Yoga And Parkinson's Disease

A Journey To Health And Healing

Peggy Van Hulsteyn
With Barbara Gage And Connie Fisher
Photographs By Jeanie Puleston Fleming, PhD

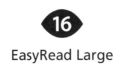

EasyRead Large

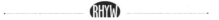

Copyright Page from the Original Book

Visit our website at www.demoshealth.com

ISBN: 978-1-936303-50-2
e-book ISBN: 978-1-61705-172-2

Acquisitions Editor: Julia Pastore
Compositor: diacriTech

Medical information provided by Demos Health, in the absence of a visit with a health care professional, must be considered as an educational service only. This book is not designed to replace a physician's independent judgment about the appropriateness or risks of a procedure or therapy for a given patient. Our purpose is to provide you with information that will help you make your own health care decisions.

The information and opinions provided here are believed to be accurate and sound, based on the best judgment available to the authors, editors, and publisher, but readers who fail to consult appropriate health authorities assume the risk of injuries. The publisher is not responsible for errors or omissions. The editors and publisher welcome any reader to report to the publisher any discrepancies or inaccuracies noticed.

Library of Congress Cataloging-in-Publication Data

Van Hulsteyn, Peggy.
  Yoga and Parkinson's disease : a journey to health and healing / Peggy van Hulsteyn, with Barbara Gage and Connie Fisher; photographs by Jeanie Puleston Fleming, PhD.
    pages cm
  Includes bibliographical references and index.
  ISBN 978-1-936303-50-2
1. Parkinson's disease–Exercise therapy. 2. Yoga–Therapeutic use. 3. Mind and body.
  I. Gage, Barbara, 1943- II. Fisher, Connie, 1948- III. Title.
  RC382.V33 2013
  616.8'330642–dc23
                              2013020954

Special discounts on bulk quantities of Demos Health books are available to corporations, professional associations, pharmaceutical companies, health care organizations, and other qualifying groups. For details, please contact:

Special Sales Department
Demos Medical Publishing, LLC
11 West 42nd Street, 15th Floor
New York, NY 10036
Phone: 800-532-8663 or 212-683-0072
Fax: 212-941-7842
E-mail: specialsales@demosmedpub.com

Printed in the United States of America by Bang Printing.
13 14 15 16 17 / 5 4 3 2 1

TABLE OF CONTENTS

Praise for Yoga and Parkinson's Disease

"In this kind and instructive book, Peggy van Hulsteyn shares her struggles with Parkinson's disease and how the practice of yoga has eased her path. With compassion, humor, and a hard fought perspective, she has written an inspiring book and seeks to provide a practical guide to others in coping with Parkinson's disease."
—U.S. Senator Tom Udall (D-NM)

"A must-read for the recently diagnosed or people at any stage of Parkinson's disease. Her practical tips and well-explained poses will help anyone with Parkinson's explore ways to live as fully as possible. Van Hulsteyn guides the reader living with the disease to view yoga as a healing practice that will increase flexibility and mobility."
—Joyce Oberdorf, president and CEO, National Parkinson Foundation

"I am inspired and enthused by van Hulsteyn's ebullient wit, humor, and positive spirit. *Yoga and Parkinson's Disease* is one of those much needed books that empowers, motivates, and educates people dealing with Parkinson's disease."

—Karl Robb, author of *A Soft Voice in a Noisy World: A Guide to Dealing and Healing with Parkinson's Disease*

"Inspiring and motivating ... a non-threatening and very practical guide to starting a yoga practice. In wonderfully witty and humorous prose, van Hulsteyn shares her story of living with Parkinson's disease and succinctly summarizes the value of exercise, particularly yoga, for dealing with the many symptoms of this disease."

—Cynthia Marie Fox, PhD, CCC-SLP, co-founder and vice president of operations of LSVT Global, Inc.

Also by Peggy van Hulsteyn

Vanity in Washington
Diary of a Santa Fe Cat
Sleeping with Literary Lions: The Booklover's
Guide to Bed and Breakfasts
The Birder's Guide to Bed and Breakfasts
What Every Business Woman Needs To Know To Get Ahead
Mind Your Own Business

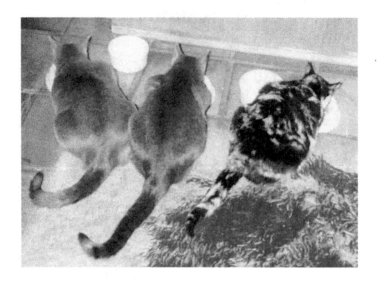

To the memory of my three beloved felines who were the embodiment of everything good about yoga:

*The brimming over with love
Apache
The elegant, dashing, and soulful
Bosque
The impish, adorable Vanity*

And to David, my soul mate, who has been with me every step of the way.

Foreword

Who should read Peggy van Hulsteyn's wonderfully witty, entertaining, and very practical guide to the practice of yoga as it pertains to the treatment of Parkinson's disease (PD)?

If you have PD and are already practicing yoga, you know how good it is for you, but in this book you will find encouragement and useful advice to help you deepen your practice. (And I forgive you if you've skipped this foreword entirely in your eagerness to jump right in!)

If you have PD and have not yet tried yoga, then my advice is this: Do not hesitate a moment before committing yourself. There is no doubt among experts that exercise is a critically important component to treatment, and I believe no less important than medication and surgery. In fact, whenever I find that a patient of mine is unsure whether to start taking medication, I counsel that the best use of medicine is to facilitate ongoing physical activity.

But what type of exercise is best for PD? The answer is the one you enjoy, because it is the one you will continue to do. Yoga is a simple and relaxing activity that will quickly demonstrate tangible benefits. Moreover, PD is a not only a disorder of movement but also one of posture. At present, no available medical treatment alone can effectively forestall the changes in posture that occur over time, but we know yoga can help. And unlike other general exercise regimens, yoga offers a way of looking at the world that can provide hope and comfort.

Who else should read this book?

The spouse, relative, or friend of a person with PD will find it to be a useful resource and an invitation to become a yoga partner. Reading these pages could be the start of a great journey together.

Healthcare professionals who see patients with PD should have a copy for their office shelf. The clear illustrations and instructions will demystify at a glance how the practice of yoga can be of benefit to clients.

And every reader will be inspired by van Hulsteyn's uplifting personal story of a travel writer's journey to a surprising territory she did not expect to be assigned to: The land of the neurologist. Her perspective on learning of her diagnosis and coming to her own terms with PD offers the kind of insight not found in any medical treatise.

Scientists and physicians on every continent, including me, have dedicated their careers to understanding the cause of PD and finding a cure. Every day we come closer to creating better medical approaches to treatment. I am sure you will find it as fascinating as I do that the next generation of treatments are being developed to affect the brain in the same positive ways exercise does. But as van Hulsteyn states "until then, there is yoga."

This doctor recommends: Get started now!

Scott J. Sherman MD, PhD
Associate Professor of Neurology
Director, Movement Disorders
The University of Arizona

Preface

If you have Parkinson's, you will need yoga.

Parkinson's disease (PD) is a movement disorder that keeps you from moving. Yoga is a 5,000-year-old practice that helps put movement back into your life.

Michael J. Fox, perhaps PD's greatest champion, calls Parkinson's "the gift that keeps on taking."

Yoga, on the other hand, is a gift that never stops giving.

Parkinson's goal is to turn you into the Tin Man!

Your goal is to have your oilcan always ready.

Yoga can be that oilcan.

Parkinson's is about rigidity, anxiety, and despair.

Yoga enhances strength, stability, balance, limberness, and calm.

Yoga teaches movement with greater ease.

Yoga embraces the philosophy that this moment is all there is.

Acknowledgments

"There is no friend as loyal as a book."

—Ernest Hemingway

I love to read and I revere books. As Anna Quindlen reminds us in *How Reading Changed My Life,* "Books are the plane, and the train, and the road. They are the destination, and the journey. They are home."

Every time I write a new book, I am filled with admiration for authors. It's an honorable profession but a difficult one.

One of the problems I had early on as a writer was the feeling of being all alone.

But on this book, I had nary a pang of loneliness. Never once during the writing of *Yoga and Parkinson's* did I feel like a recluse. Au contraire. It may take a village to raise a child, but writing this book seemed to take several small countries. As a matter of fact, I often felt like the director of a small independent film.

The closest I got to a red carpet moment, however, was buying a pair of red yoga pants. But in that Academy award vein, I have a long list of people to thank.

So, the envelope, please.

Because I am fresh out of Oscars, I will express my gratitude in yoga parlance:

A Warrior Pose for courage to my yoga consultants, who were advisors, teachers, and friends:

Barbara Gage and Connie Fisher

"Namaste."

A Sun Salutation of appreciation to The Medical Dream Team, all compassionate and sensitive physicians who, in spite of a broken medical system, have remained whole:

Paul Gordon, MD
Scott Sherman, MD
Claire Henchcliffe, MD

A Breath of Joy posture celebrating long-standing and outstanding teachers, who were gracious enough to give to me, and thus you, some incredible tips:

John Argue
Lori Newell
Cynthia Fox, PhD
Angela and Karl Robb

The Lion Pose for Technical Support, par excellence:

Sasha Mahar, my wonderful, logical assistant who kept me organized, edited, amused, and sane.

Jeanie Puleston Fleming, my first-rate photographer who excels at everything she tries.

Tim Nagy, the magic computer tamer.

Michelle Schumacher, photographer extraordinaire of Miss Isabel.

A fluttering Butterfly Pose to Friends who became my Readers:

Mary Gay Rogers
Valerie Brooker
Elaine Pinkerton Coleman
Jann Arrington Wolcott
Pam Cully

A Mountain Pose, for strength and sturdiness, to:

Jeanne Nolan for getting the ball rolling. Meredith Machen for matchmaking.

Robb Foster for encouragement and insight.

Timothy Bowden, PhD, and Diane Bowden, good friends and all-round cheerleaders.

Kim Rubin, for sharing her PD journey.

A graceful Cat Pose for the feline flexibility of the superb models: Diane Bowden, Tim Bowden, Joleen Racque Frank, Peter Hagen, Philip Nichols, Donna Kidby, Sarah Schumacher, Isabel Shumacher, Carol Price, Barbara Gage, Connie Fisher, and David van Hulsteyn, PhD.

A tip of the yoga mat to the wonderful people at Demos Health: Julia Pastore, Beth Kaufman Barry, and Lee Oglesby. All were top notch in every way.

Author's Note

It has been said that, "When you're ready, the teacher you need appears before you."

I must have been more than ready, for when I needed a yoga advisor for this book, two appeared. This plethora of yoga teachers was a boon to this project, and the combined forces of two lifelong yoga devotees have made it a far more enjoyable process for me. Each yogi contributed her own brand of insight, wisdom, creativity, and humor.

Researching this book has kept me extremely active. Twice a week for many years, I have been attending the lovely class of my Kripalu trained yoga teacher, Barbara Gage. Her guidance has anchored me through many trials and adventures. It was this practice that inspired me to write about how helpful yoga is in dealing with Parkinson's disease.

Not long after I began writing this book, Connie Fisher appeared on my doorstep, offering to give me a weekly private class. Connie was working on her masters degree in Iyengar Yoga Therapy and needed a few more credits to complete the course. It was the best of symbiotic relations: she saw me as extra credit, and I saw her as a pleasant and efficient way to exercise. I always wanted to be on the top floor of the television series *Upstairs, Downstairs,* so I liked the concept of a yoga teacher who made house calls.

In my fantasy of being part of the British aristocracy, exclusive home visitations were right up there with high tea. And in my imaginary PBS production, Connie could have easily played the role of the enigmatic, windswept English village character. She was always a breath of fresh air, riding over on her bike, armed with her yoga backpack, upbeat attitude, and Thoreau-like lifestyle of "simplify, simplify." She was like a haiku poem come to life.

ABOUT THE AUTHOR

Peggy van Hulsteyn, who has practiced yoga for over 40 years, was diagnosed with Parkinson's disease 12 years ago. She has since become a Parkinson's advocate and writes extensively on this subject. Her feature article describing how yoga can benefit people with Parkinson's was presented in both the American and Chinese versions of *Yoga Journal.*

During her career, van Hulsteyn was assistant travel editor of *Mademoiselle* magazine in New York City, southeastern director of publicity for American International Pictures in Atlanta, owner of an award-winning advertising agency in Austin, and advertising lecturer at the University of Texas. Van Hulsteyn won the Southwest Writers Workshop Storyteller Award for Best Novel for her murder mystery in progress. She was awarded first place for nonfiction by the New Mexico Press Women for her book *Mind Your Own Business,* and she won a Certificate of Excellence in Humor for *Vanity in*

Washington from the Cat Writers' Association.

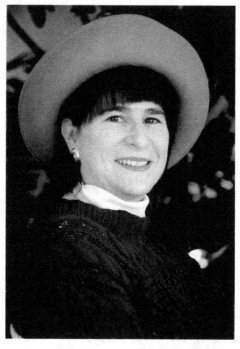

Photo by Tim Thompson

She has written for *Mademoiselle, Cosmopolitan, Modern Bride, Country Living, Cat Fancy, New Mexico Magazine, American Way (American Airlines in-flight magazine),* and newspapers such as the *Washington Post,* the *Los Angeles Times,* the *Miami Herald,* the *Kansas City Star,* the *Chicago Tribune,* the *San Francisco Examiner,* and *USA Today.* Her work has been translated into Japanese, Spanish, Dutch, and

Portuguese and has appeared in Australian periodicals.

Van Hulsteyn, who attended the University of Missouri Journalism School, holds a degree in English and journalism from Indiana University. She divides her time between Santa Fe, New Mexico, and Tucson, Arizona, with her physicist husband and is currently working on a mystery and another Vanity the Cat book. She and her husband are hoping to be adopted by some kittens soon.

Visit her at www.pdhatlady.com

ABOUT THE YOGA CONSULTANTS

Barbara Gage is a certified Kripalu Yoga teacher, who did intense yoga teacher's training at the Kripalu Yoga Institute in Lenox, Massachusetts, in 1982 and advanced yoga teacher's training in 1990. Her classes feature the classical yoga postures, meditation, breathing practices, and reading from the Sanskrit texts. She has been a yoga teacher for 35 years. Gage is a respected psychotherapist in private practice in Santa Fe, New Mexico, and a recognized photographer specializing in nature photography. She has a BA in social work from Eckerd College, St. Petersburg, Florida, and an MA in counseling from the University of New Mexico in Albuquerque.

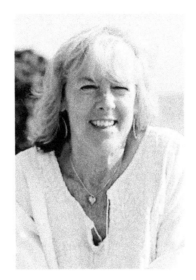

Photo by Howard Steven Gross

For further information, visit www.barbaragage.com

Connie Fisher has traveled the world with an interest in things Asian/Oriental. After a trip to China and two trips to India, she returned to study yoga with Gary Kraftsow, founder of the American Viniyoga Institute. She is a doctor of Oriental medicine, a massage therapist, and since 2008, a Viniyoga instructor. Her life has been devoted to the study of the human body. In 2012, she became certified in yoga therapy from the American Viniyoga Institute in California.

She has been a professional ski instructor in Santa Fe, New Mexico, and Aspen, Colorado, and was one of the first women on the Aspen Ski Patrol. In spare moments, she may be at a film festival or hiking in the mountains. Fisher now lives in Seattle, where she practices yoga with her twin sister, her next-door neighbor, who in turn is teaching her to garden.

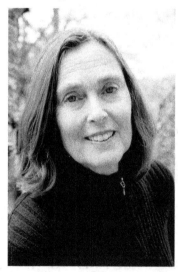

Photo by Bill Thorness

ABOUT THE PHOTOGRAPHER

The photos of Jeanie Puleston Fleming, PhD, have appeared in publications such as *Travel & Leisure, Food & Wine,* the *New York Times,* the *International Herald Tribune, New Mexico Magazine,* and the *Albuquerque Journal,* and as illustrations for the book *Zozobra* (University of New Mexico Press).

She has a PhD in French and teaches lively French classes in Santa Fe. She has a peripatetic lifestyle and can often be found at her home in Provence, France, or traveling the world with her hydrologist husband.

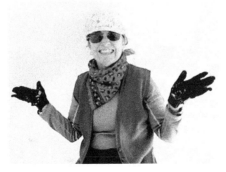

Photo by Jeanie Puleston Fleming

PART I

YOGA TO THE RESCUE

1

My Story

Learn from yesterday, live for today, hope for tomorrow. The important thing is not to stop questioning.
—Albert Einstein

When mortality tapped me on the shoulder 12 years ago, it was a transforming moment—a sea change, a lightning bolt, an epiphany.

My world turned upside down when I heard the life-changing words, "You have Parkinson's disease." I didn't hear another word the neurologist said. All I could hear was the word "Parkinson's" rolling around in my mind like a crashing wave on a sea wall.

My malady had begun as numbness, a stiffness on my left side, particularly my left hand. In my case, I never even considered Parkinson's disease (PD). I had convinced myself that I had carpal tunnel, an inconvenient but kind of cool occupational handicap. I was already wearing a brace on my stiff left arm. Talk about an author's hubris! I had the notion that signing too many copies of my latest book had caused this affliction. Wishful thinking; I am right handed.

My husband, David, and I traveled to Denver for an appointment with a noted neurologist. What she wasn't noted for, we discovered, was her humanity.

While waiting seemingly forever in her freezing office to find what a magnetic resonance imaging (MRI) brain scan revealed, I, by force of habit, turned to the warmth and familiarity of my 40-year yoga practice. I began to meditate and imagined I was at one of my favorite places in the world, a wildlife refuge in New Mexico called the Bosque del Apache. As I deeply inhaled the cool air, I watched the sunrise over the wetlands, magically turning the black sky a vivid red-orange. A flock of sandhill cranes, flying in V-formation, whooshed overhead. I took some cleansing breaths and chanted my go-to mantra, *namaste*, over and over.

I came plummeting back to reality moments later when I heard the words "brain tumor." The doctor, who reminded me of an unsavory character from a Dickens novel, displayed my MRI. "Initially, a brain tumor was indicated, but I've ruled out this possibility," she said. She was visibly disappointed by this conclusion, and that disappointment morphed into downright boredom when she matter-of-factly dubbed my elusive ailment as the mysterious arm. When she gave me the diagnostic assignment of putting pegs in a board with first my left hand, then my right, the clouds lifted.

In a monotone voice, she announced, "You have Parkinson's disease."

I was in shock. After mentally reeling for a moment, my robust imagination sprang to my defense. Desperately, I told myself the woman was clearly a mountebank like the fake doctor in the movie, *Catch Me If You Can.* Or else she was stark raving mad.

David's face registered complete disbelief, but being of the English school of optimism, he tried to find something positive to hang onto. An exercise enthusiast—some, like me, would say a fanatic—he asked the doctor if exercise might help.

"Try it, if you like," she replied briskly, "but I doubt that it will make any difference." She showed us the door so she could dash to a hospital meeting.

She was completely wrong of course.

Luckily, I soon met other doctors and specialists who encouraged me to continue with my yoga, and in the 12 years since my diagnosis, I have found it to be invaluable. And I am not alone.

My hope is that, with this book, you will also experience the benefits of a regular yoga practice.

As a journalist, I always prepare for interviews, and none was more important than the first one I had with a neurologist whose specialty is PD.

What is a neurologist anyway? I've heard it whispered that they are the Brahmins of the medical caste system and speak a secret language known as Medicalese.

Research was clearly called for, so I rang up a college roommate whose second marriage was to one of these mysterious creatures. I had never met Husband Number Two; when I asked my chum to describe the general breed, she started laughing.

"You ought to know better than anyone what neurologists are like; they have the same DNA as physicists. You wrote the definitive quote about physicists; I have it stitched in needlepoint. It's priceless."

Indeed, for a mystery I am working on, I wrote: "The breed known as the physicist is an interesting blend of geek, genius, absent-minded professor and wonder-struck little boy."

"So," said my old companion from long-ago journalism school days, "you've got your own translator to take along to this first meeting."

"It's true," I said, making some inane comment about the smallness of the cosmos.

But she was right. I was indeed related to one of this tribe: My husband, a PhD physicist at Los Alamos National Laboratory, who always ends his love poems with one of Maxwell's equations.

So, armed with my reporter's notebook and my scientific guide, I bravely made the intimidating journey to the unknown physician's office.

As a quick aside, it's worthwhile from the beginning to invest the time and energy to select the right doctor; this is an important relationship in long-term diseases like PD where the doctor–patient bond becomes a "sacred trust." Always look for a sense of simpatico, a feeling I value in my relationship with my current neurologist, Scott Sherman, MD, PhD, and which I also experienced immediately upon meeting my first Parkinson's neurologist, Dr. Paul Gordon.

You can tell a lot about a person by his office. Dr. Gordon's looked just like him—attractive, welcoming, and well-organized. The Navajo rugs, Indian pots, handsome leather chairs, and a floor-to-ceiling library blended perfectly with a black and brown set of monogrammed doctor's bags, which artfully shared a shelf with a collection of African sculpture. Tucked between the African sculpture and the doctor's bags, barely visible to the human eye, was a rolled up yoga mat.

Eureka! I liked this doctor already. We had something important in common. I was ready with my first question.

While I fished through my purse for my notebook, the two members of the same tribe got acquainted as boys in science are wont to do. David threw out a few hard science questions, and although much of it sounded like Sanskrit to me, the moods of the players were jocular and the conversation flowed. Then there was the "guy thing," the other club most men are devoted to—*sports.* David tossed Paul a few baseball questions, which he answered with aplomb.

The initiation ritual was over, and I could safely get to the mission at hand.

"I noted that you have a yoga mat hidden neatly in your office," I said tentatively. "I've taken yoga for almost 30 years."

"Then you're ahead of the game in dealing with Parkinson's," he said with a winning smile. "Exercise is a key component in the battle against PD, and in my opinion, a gentle Hatha yoga practice is the best all-round physical activity there is. I do yoga every day."

He won me over with the affirming, "I'm impressed with your eyesight and powers of observation; that yoga mat is miniscule."

I smiled coyly and thought to myself, "This doctor is authentic. He talks the talk and does the yoga. He's the poster child for his profession—trim, fit, and almost zen-like in his demeanor."

Paul Gordon remained my doctor for years. He is calm and meditative and speaks in simple phrases that are clear, precise, and easy to understand. After lo these many years of speaking to a gaggle of neurologists, I have dubbed Paul Gordon the "patient's doctor."

Below is a Q&A session we had covering the basics of PD:

Q. What exactly is PD?

A. PD is a neurodegenerative disease. This means that, for some reason we don't yet understand, a group of nerve cells in the *substantia nigra* region of the brain die off too soon or degenerate. With PD, it happens that the group of cells that die are the ones that produce dopamine.

Q. What is dopamine?

A. Dopamine is the neurotransmitter molecule that helps us to move quickly and automatically. When you have PD, less dopamine is produced. By the time patients develop symptoms, they are producing 70 percent less dopamine than normal.

Q. Am I going to die from this?

A. No one dies from Parkinson's, they die with it. In other words, people with Parkinson's die from the same things as everybody else—heart disease, pneumonia, or some other ailment.

Q. Will I end up in a nursing home?

A. Most of our patients don't go anywhere near a nursing home. Many people with Parkinson's have indomitable spirits and go on with their lives despite their disabilities. For example, I have a patient who can't walk anymore, yet doesn't want to give up cultivating her crops, so she works on her hands and knees every day in her garden. I have another patient who lives in a small farming community and gets around her property to feed her animals with the help of guide ropes. These are enduring people.

Q. It sounds as if having a positive, can-do attitude is an important component in hanging on to your quality of life. Am I right?

A. Absolutely. There are physical limitations, sometimes severe ones, but patients with determination and optimism can still lead quality lives.

Q. What about dementia? I think I could handle being physically disabled better than not being able to think or remember.

A. The majority of Parkinson's people I see don't have trouble with memory or mental functioning. We are finding that having an education and mental activity helps compensate for anatomical changes. It's becoming increasingly clear that lack of education may result in less cognitive reserve.

Q. So general recommendations for keeping the mind alert—such as learning a new language, reading, and taking classes—apply to people with Parkinson's?

A. What I have seen with my patients is if they have an unbridled passion that overrides everything, it makes a big difference. It helps if there is a goal tied in with this passion. You're a good example of how this works—with your books, speeches, and deadlines. Your mind is in good shape.

Q. What about a cure?

A. There are great scientists working on promising projects that could lead to a cure. However, there is a problem with the funding of these grants. The National Institutes of Health, which used to fund much of the scientific research in the United States, has drastically cut money for basic research. It's hard to explain to my patients how this country was able to fund two wars, yet can't pay for research to cure Parkinson's. But, despite this funding problem, the research continues.

Q. I know that you are a fellow at the Hôpital de la Pitié-Salpêtrière in Paris. Can you tell us about breakthroughs in brain research?

A. Brain research is the last great frontier of medicine. We are trying to learn why brain cells don't regenerate.

If you cut your finger, the skin grows back and heals; however, for reasons we don't understand, when brain cells are damaged they fail to grow back. But we are on the brink of discovery. Ever since the first medication for PD was prescribed in the late 1800s, there has been only symptomatic treatment for the disease. Today, we are embarking on a generation of research designed to develop disease-altering medications—medicines that will slow the progress of Parkinson's as we move toward the cure.

Q. Discuss the complexity of the brain.

A. I am still in awe of the complexity of the brain. The frontal lobes make us human. It's what makes Peggy able to write a good sentence or put together a sophisticated outfit. It is what makes David able to do complicated equations and write papers on magnetoencephalography.

Q. While waiting for the cure, what do you recommend that patients like me do?

A. View your diagnosis as an impetus to get into the best physical and mental shape possible. Identify all that is meaningful to you. Make the most of every day. And do your yoga.

David and I remain in touch with Paul (now a neurologist at the northern Navajo Medical Center in Shiprock, New Mexico) and once in a while catch up over a leisurely brunch in Santa Fe. Always, his first question is, "Are you keeping up with your yoga?"

My yoga practice has spanned four decades, through wildly different times and places. Despite the variety, yoga has always accommodated my needs, providing a perfectly calibrated counterpoint to each phase of my life.

I was a young bride when I discovered yoga in 1970. After a brief and passionate courtship, I had married David, a dynamic college professor. Shortly afterward, we moved to Austin, Texas, where he had secured a faculty position at the university. I embraced marriage and my new family with gusto, creating a home and receiving on-the-job training from my husband's two young children. I taught myself how to cook via the books of Julia Child. I gained knowledge about France, I gained cooking skills, and I gained 10 pounds. I organized dinner parties and wine tastings with my newfound vibrant community.

My pursuits weren't merely domestic, however. In addition to exploring and enjoying life in my stimulating new hometown, I was active in the Women's Rights Movement. And, in a time and place where it was unusual for a woman to own a business, I decided to partner with two former coworkers and open an ad agency, which won accolades and awards for its innovations.

My energy was boundless, and in yoga class, I found the rare opportunity to slow down and relax. I left each class feeling refreshed and renewed. I loved how yoga toned my body, but I was riveted by the spiritual rejuvenation it offered. Under the guidance of my yoga teacher, I began reading books on yoga, spirituality, and meditation, another practice I continue to this day.

My yoga and reading practices were a much needed anchor during the next phase of my life. David had obtained a position at the Los Alamos National

Laboratory, so we relocated to Santa Fe, New Mexico.

The town was a culture shock. My New York City personality ("Are we there yet?") did not match the laid-back *mañana* style of mellow Santa Fe.

Although a cultural mecca, laden with a rich history of science (birth of the nuclear age) and art (from rock art to pop art, from Aztec to high tech), Santa Fe was still the slowest place I'd ever been, so laid back I felt I had been laid under! I had what the Navajo call the "hurry sickness," and could not figure out why this town seemed to move at ice-age glacial speed. I wanted things done in a "New York minute," while Santa Fe, dubbed the "City Different," thought otherwise. Guess who won?

When I saw an advertisement for a yoga class led by a psychotherapist from Chicago, I leapt at the chance to attend, hoping any discussion in class would be intense and snappy. I was not disappointed—Pam, the yoga teacher, was charming, friendly, funny, and, like me, brand new to town. We bonded immediately.

Because the class was held in the late afternoon in Pam's home, we would often stay for a potluck supper. We used to joke that we had to stay there because no one could remember how to get out. Like most Santa Fe homes then, it was a tiny house with no address, on a street with no name. In vintage Santa Fe, directions to a party often included a folksy expression like "Turn right at the sleeping calico cat."

This yoga class provided not only practice, but community—a network of sympathetic souls who supported and challenged each other. Increasing our skills, we deepened our downward dogs and performed show-off headstands. Yoga gained an athletic dimension as I tested the vitality and suppleness of my body in a way I never had before. Growing up in Indiana in the 1950s, when little girls wore dresses with sashes, and Title 9 was in a future far, far away, I had never been encouraged to engage in any sport. Now I found myself capable of heretofore unimaginable feats! It was intoxicating to watch my strength and flexibility grow, and I gained a newfound appreciation for my body.

My yoga group, with the help of reading the works of the Dalai Lama and Thich Nhat Hanh, helped me make the quantum professional leap from the adrenaline rush of advertising to the slower, more reflective world of author and teacher. Even now, patience is not one of my virtues. However, I am very grateful that I was forced to switch gears. This is the eighth book I have written, and I have enjoyed them all. Had I not moved to Santa Fe and pursued yoga, I would probably not be listed in the card catalogue in the Library of Congress. Thank you, Yoga. Gracias, La Villa Real de la Santa Fé de San Francisco de Asís.

My Parkinson's diagnosis once again shifted yoga's meaning and impact in my life. Distressed and distracted, contemplating a newly foreboding future, I was regularly shuttling among various specialists as I learned a new and dreadful language of symptoms and medications. I threw myself into my writing projects, finding work provided structure and familiarity to a newly chaotic and alien life. During this turmoil, my yoga practice became more sporadic. I tried to explain to David my growing symptoms and how exiled I felt from myself. Words had always tripped wittily off my tongue, but now I would be disrupted by the occasional stammer, and I would unexpectedly stumble when I wanted to prance. I felt possessed. During an early spring day when my symptoms were especially disorienting, I sought the warmth of our sunlit garden and struck a Warrior Pose. A wave of relief came over me as my muscles obediently flowed into the familiar position, one of my old favorites. I felt restored to myself. That moment has stayed with me, and I have ever since turned to yoga to keep connected with myself.

Resuming my yoga practice was even more of a challenge since my PD progressed. At first I felt as if I was starring in my own private version of *The Invasion of the Body Snatchers*. I became a character from *The Twilight Zone.* My body perception grew increasingly disoriented. My walk became more tentative and deliberate.

I began losing motor control. My stiff left arm was not budging. And my voice was off on its own little holiday. I had never had a strong voice; now I was the ghost whisperer.

Yoga has made an enormous difference. Physically, it helps me to build strength, stability, balance, and limberness. Emotionally, it calms me. And intellectually, it stimulates me, boosting my creativity. "Yoga builds confidence," as Dr. Becky Farley, a neuroscientist and researcher at the University of Arizona, once told me. "When people embrace yoga, they become more relaxed and able to control tremors, become more balanced and generally feel better about themselves."

Emotionally, yoga is my sanctuary, retreat, and meditation chamber. There's comfort and peace in that no matter what is going on in the outside world, the yoga postures remain blissfully the same.

The Cat Pose, one of my favorites, looks exactly like the elegant stretch performed daily by one of my beloved felines and always loosens the

Parkinson-induced rigidity of my back and entire left side; the stiffness is replaced with a little bit of a cat swagger.

Child's Pose brings a general feeling of relaxation and well-being.

Warrior Pose bids me to focus on personal courage. As I bend my right knee and lift my arms to shoulder length, I truly feel like a heroic warrior and mentally pat myself on the back for being so courageous in my daily battle with PD. It's a heady feeling that lasts long after the class is over.

The Breath of Joy Pose opens me up, and I feel gratitude for all the many blessings I still have in my life.

During the meditations and poses, I get back in touch with the playful, childlike part of me that had become lost in the serious, grown-up world of coping with Parkinson's. It was at the end of a yoga class that I came up with my favorite writing project—using my real life cat, Vanity, as the heroine of a series of gentle satires.

The relaxation and flow of yoga class often boosts my creativity and gets my juices going. Ideas bubble up and dance across my mind, so I always keep a notebook ready. I use the word "flow" intentionally. In his book, *Flow: The Psychology of Optimal Experience,* psychologist Mihaly Csíkszentmihályi sets forth the theory that people are most happy when they are in flow—a state of complete focus with the activity at hand. During flow one is so absorbed in an activity that nothing else seems to matter. Csíkszentmihályi claims that engaging in a sense of flow on a regular basis encourages a positive attitude and more contented life. Yoga and meditation are prominent in the list of activities he says promote flow. Time and again, I have experienced respite from the trying circumstances of PD while practicing yoga.

When I was first diagnosed with PD, it seemed as if mortality was calling me every five minutes. This Mortality Gal was a big pest; she was reminiscent of all the annoying phone calls that are so jarring during political campaigns. You know the type—ceaseless hecklers who make you want to throw all your telephones into the nearest mountain stream.

And the old crone had no sense of humor—she appeared to be the third cousin, twice removed, of the grim reaper. Every symptom or doctor's report was another chilling ring on the black phone. I did everything I could to keep it at bay—I ignored it, I denied it, I shouted, "You've got the wrong number!" and hung up the phone. Despite all my efforts, the bell kept ringing to beat the band.

Mortality has been calling for 12 years now. During this time, I have learned not only to listen to her message, but also to appreciate it. To be sure, it is a wake-up call, but instead of alerting me to pending doom, I have found it to be an unexpected cheerleader. For, once I listened to what she had to say, I realized it's not death on the line, but life. And life calls me to dive deep into the Carpe Diem pool.

"Don't postpone joy," she reminds me.

"That novel is not going to write itself," she warns.

"That exotic trip you were going to take in the future should be planned for the day after tomorrow," she orders.

I am happy to report that I am taking her advice. I just plunked down the cash I was planning to put into a savings account to whisk my husband off for a romantic sojourn. I don't wait for Christmas to give presents to friends; I bestow them all year round.

I threw a spectacular Nancy Drew birthday party for my chum, Val, complete with costumes and a comfort-food dinner from *The Nancy Drew Cookbook;* of course, I got to play "the girl detective."

No matter what I am doing, I put it away when Isabel, my lively and beautiful great-granddaughter comes over and wants to play. Isabel, age 5, who has been taking yoga for over a year, teaches me how to be in the moment. This precocious charmer leads me in a spontaneous yoga class; with the potency of the ancient power of this practice on our side, we mighty van Hulsteyn women keep this insistent disease at bay.

In this new "Seize the Moment" regimen, I remind my husband of over 40 years that he's never been sexier than when he's bringing me my morning dose of Parkinson's medicine (before these pills kick in, it's difficult to walk).

By writing and lecturing about Parkinson's, as well as campaigning for more funding for Parkinson's research, I'm searching for meaning and a sense of purpose in my diagnosis. I know that my mortality is always out there, ready to dial my number, and that her message is that I should fill my life with as much laughter, whimsy, and joy as possible. I strive to view life as a glass all the way full. As Viktor E. Frankl, concentration camp survivor and professor of neurology at the University of Vienna, reminds us in *Man's Search for Meaning:* "It is not the events in our lives that determine who we become, but the meaning we choose to place on those events."

I urge you to see the meaning of this hardship as a call to crown yourself reigning royal over your precious life, to gather your roses and your friends, practice yoga every day, cultivate your garden, hug your cat, learn French, read *Auntie Mame* to your niece, and embrace its message to "Live, live, live!"

2

Research and Findings on Yoga for Parkinson's Disease

Medical research in the twentieth century mostly takes place in the lab; in the Renaissance, though, researchers went first and foremost to the library to see what the ancients had said.
—Peter Lewis Allen

I am happy to say that during the course of writing this book, I was inspired by the breadth and depth of work that has been devoted to the benefits of exercise in general and yoga in particular for people like me who suffer from Parkinson's disease (PD). Until a cure for this insidious disease is developed, we will have to rely upon any or all of the therapies that are available to help us slow its progress. The options may include physical exercise or music therapy or vocal projection, but because yoga has been part of my life for as long as I can remember, this is where my passion lies.

In order to take full advantage of yoga's healing power, I felt I owed it to myself and to others to find out just what it is that makes the practice work for me. To this end I have done extensive research on the subject and am pleased to share my findings with you. I am also including here information and recommendations of individuals who have been dealing with the subject for many years. The support and encouragement I received from Lori Newell, Dr. Claire Henchcliffe, and John Argue have made this book come alive for me as I hope it will for you.

According to a finding by the Parkinson Foundation of the National Capital Area, "Recent research has shown that yoga is a powerful complementary therapy for neurological diseases like PD. Yoga is a great way to exercise the mind and body. It also helps to improve body strength."

A more academic study, performed by researchers at the John F. Kennedy Institute in Denmark, describes how "Using 11C-raclopride PET we demonstrated increased endogenous dopamine release in the ventral striatum during Yoga Nidra meditation.... During meditation, 11C-raclopride binding in ventral striatum decreased by 7.9%. This corresponds to a 65% increase in endogenous dopamine release."

These observations indicate that yoga appears to offer benefits to Parkinson's sufferers not only during the exercise phase but during the meditative phase as well. Jeannette Macturk, a Britain-based yoga teacher who specialized in yoga for PD, wrote, "I appreciate the better quality of life the practice of Yoga offers. Learning to control the breath, practicing movements to keep the body supple and stilling the mind through relaxation, are all helpful towards a healthy and happy lifestyle."

According to Dr. Nina Browner, clinical director of Movement Disorders at the University of North Carolina at Chapel Hill:

There is a growing body of evidence regarding the benefits of exercise in terms of neuroplasticity and the ability of the brain to self repair. Studies with 6-hydroxydopamine animal models of PD have found that exercise has protective benefits against the onset of PD symptoms, possibly due to the release of so called "trophic factors" and greater cerebral oxygenation, which together promote new cell growth and cell survival.

Guide4Living, an online self-help organization that promotes alternative treatments, states:

Yoga improves flexibility, strength and balance and it can give Parkinson's disease sufferers better posture. People who practice yoga and/or meditation report feeling less stressed and having a sense of psychological well-being. In a Parkinson's Disease Society survey on complementary therapies, yoga and meditation were rated the most beneficial with 95% of participants reporting some improvement in their symptoms.

Lori Newell, author of *The Book Of Exercise and Yoga For Those With Parkinson's Disease,* explains the correlation between exercise and PD in the following way:

> While exercise cannot cure this disease, it can improve your lung capacity, muscle strength, balance, gait, the ability to initiate movement and flexibility. Exercise can lift your spirits, improve everyday functioning and help you to feel less victimized by your condition. The practice of yoga can help improve balance, increase flexibility, and reduce stress. The goal of yoga is to become more connected with your body and mind through the use of movement, breath work and meditation.

Claire Henchcliffe, MD, DPhil, director of the PD and Movements Disorders Institute at Weill Cornell Medical College, conducted a pilot study at Cornell University that placed 15 people with Parkinson's in 10 week-long yoga programs. She observed that the participants reported less stiffness, better sleep, and wellness and notes that:

> A surprising side effect was the social support the class provided ... a lot hinges on sharing problems that doctors don't have firsthand experience with. At a support group, people get first-hand information and become proactive ... After a pilot study on the effects of yoga on PD back in 2005 ended, the class lived on. It's been going strong since. Many of my patients remain enthusiastic practitioners and are convinced yoga helps them. They can learn from each other. Sometimes we doctors just need to step out of the way.

John Argue, author of *Parkinson's & the Art of Healing*, has taught movement technique to people with Parkinson's for more than three decades. During my interview with him, he enthusiastically reported that:

> People with PD should have weekly Parkinson's exercise classes for the rest of their lives, or until a cure is found. The "small group"

approach is by far the best for many reasons. Regular exercise can prevent the gradual deterioration of posture and even restore use to neglected motor functions. Exercise and training for inevitable falls can keep the strength and flexibility needed to protect a person from severe injuries.

Since "movement memory" is precisely the part of the brain that is compromised in PD, lessons will need to be reinforced over and over again. Class membership in a small group brings fellowship and relief from the stress felt in "normal" settings. Weekly classes allow people to take up multiple challenges one at a time. And weekly classes provide respite for the caregiver; the benefits of such respites cannot be exaggerated. Finally, the person and the family acquire a sense of purpose in fighting back against Parkinson's.

Just coming to the class helps all of us. The people who come to my class are the ones who have refused to let PD get the better of them. They are a self-selected group of courageous people. They are very good company indeed; they meet their challenges with humor and compassion for each other. For 27 years and counting, these are the people whose company I have had the privilege to share.

3

How to Use This Book

Whenever I feel the need to exercise, I lie down until it goes away.
—Robert Maynard Hutchins

Put no pressure on yourself; having Parkinson's disease (PD) is pressure enough. This book is to be thought of as a time-out, and the word "should" is henceforth banished. There are myriad exercises in this book, and it is entirely up to you how many you'd like to enjoy:

You can do 1.
You can do 10.
You can do 100.

You don't have to start at the very beginning. Start with the posture with the most appeal. Then check in with yourself. Do you feel like doing more or going back to bed? It's your body, your book, your time. You can do what you want. "PD affects each person differently. You are the best judge of what feels right for your body," affirms movement specialist and author Lori Newell.

Start from where you are, no matter where that might be.

Are your meds not working?

Are you experiencing so many ons and offs that you feel like a light switch?

Are you immobile?

If your body is particularly resistant to movement at this time, head immediately to Chapter 10, "Meditation."

PRACTICAL TIPS FOR BEGINNING YOUR YOGA PRACTICE

What to Wear

There are at least two schools of thought:

On one hand, "beware of all activities which require new clothes." Henry David Thoreau was the first to warn other men of the dangers of shopping. My husband still has the perfect jacket he got at Filene's Department Store in Boston when he was 19 (he's now 78). That jacket has been to 12 countries, countless parties, a concert or two. And to many a yoga class.

On the other hand, I'm an accomplished material girl who has a major in Retail Therapy. I love to shop, and yoga outfits these days are beautiful, inexpensive, and your way to spruce up the planet.

Whatever your personal philosophy on yoga attire might be, it is advised that you:
Wear loose-fitting, comfortable clothes.
Practice yoga in bare feet whenever you can.

Equipment

Use a nonslip yoga mat.

Have some pillows ready to put under your head, hips, or anywhere else you might need support.

A light, soft blanket to cover yourself during the longer, still poses.

A stable chair to use as support or for seated poses.

Glass of water.

Tissues.

Choosing a Space

Choose a dedicated space in your home where you'll always work out.

Make it as comfortable, inviting, and useful as it can possibly be.

Place everything you'll need for your practice right there, including a bottle of water and a box of tissues, and when you're finished, leave it there for the next day.

Choosing a Time

Pick a time of day when you feel your best.

Dedicate a certain amount of time each day to your workout. This can be as little as 10 minutes.

Do what you can in the time you have.

Developing a Routine

Exercise at a regular time and regular place.

Mark your exercise session on your calendar.

Always start the exercises on the same side of the body.

Staying on Track

Keep a list of why exercise is important, and look at it frequently. My list includes something my trainer, Robb, once told me: "Exercise is to PD what insulin is to diabetes." Besides, exercise—especially yoga—is good for the immune system.

Set achievable goals for your workout. For example, keep it simple. Try to hold a pose for 2 or 3 seconds longer this week. Increase the time of your class by 5 minutes; if you are really tired, roll over and do the meditations for these extra 5 minutes.

Be proud of yourself. Give yourself lots of kudos for just showing up and even more for doing such a great job!!

Don't ask yourself to do too much. "Don't defeat yourself by working too hard," suggests Parkinson's movement specialist John Argue. "If you make the exercise grueling, you may develop an aversion to it."

Keep a journal or record of your accomplishments and efforts. Recognize any changes in tightness, range of motion, or energy levels. Acknowledge your improvements.

Exercise with someone. You can encourage each other. A few "atta girls" and "good job" can work wonders.

Does the following scenario sound familiar? It's time for your solo yoga class to start. Your back hurts. Your toes are curled under. And didn't you hear on last night's forecast that it might snow today? So you put on your Scarlett O'Hara pajamas vowing to "think about it tomorrow" and crawl back into bed.

Now think of how this scene would play out if your friend Suzanne were coming over to do yoga with you. You would grumble, of course, be stiff as a board, but you would make the effort to get out of bed, prepare the yoga area, and maybe even make some tea. Having a buddy system forces you to do it; it's so easy to slack off if it's just you.

If you fall off track, start again the very next day. "Forgive yourself," counsels Argue. "Don't be too hard on yourself. Try not to build up an 'exercise debt' because you were not able to do your planned workout on any particular day. The burden of guilt may make you resentful and sulky, so just turn that debt loose. Start each day with a clean slate by forgiving yourself for not doing enough the day before. Do for today what you can for today. Forgive yourself, begin again. As the poet Rilke said, 'Always be beginning.'"

Reward yourself. Positive rewards are much more effective than punitive measures. Or as Argue puts it, "Extrinsic rewards can be very helpful in keeping that interior part of us showing up for the workout hour. So always reward yourself for your workout achievement. Think of some special treat."

For me, the word "reward" means shopping for new yoga finery. So what does the term "reward" mean to you?

Sneaking off to a movie in the middle of the day?

Treating yourself to a delicious meal at your favorite restaurant?

Visiting a new art gallery or museum?

Reading a new book or an old favorite?

Eating a small package of the best chocolates you can find? (This is not only a reward; it's an antioxidant!)

Decide for yourself, and make rewards a regular part of your routine.

Just Do It

Some days my pills haven't kicked in. Some days I have allergies. Most days I haven't gotten enough sleep. But no matter how I feel before yoga, I always feel better afterwards. The endorphins kick in, and it feels as if I have more dopamine flowing about.

The after-yoga exercise glow is comparable to one of my favorite sayings about writing, attributed to both Dorothy Parker and Gloria Steinem: "I hate writing. I like having written."

How to Choose the Right Class

I have been attending the same yoga class for the last 15 years, and one of the joys it has provided is the lovely acceptance I'm given by the other members of the class.

Use word of mouth to find a class tailor-made for your needs.

Ask other friends with Parkinson's disease or check out local PD Associations and support group websites.

If possible, find a class specifically for people with PD. It's helpful if the teacher has worked with people with PD before.

Arrange a brief interview with the teacher, or ask if you could visit one of her classes. You could stand or sit behind the class and watch. Talk to other students to find out how they feel about the class.

Or arrange for a private class to see if you and the teacher are a good fit.

Considerations:

How long is the class?

Where is it located? Is there handicapped or adequate parking? Good lighting?

How difficult is it to get through the door?

Does it address your needs?

Does it emphasize flexibility, suppleness, stability, balance, limberness, and calm?

How about meditations and inspiring readings?

NOTES ON SAFETY AND COMFORT

Within a yoga class, you have the benefit of an instructor who can guide and correct your poses. However, no expert can replace your own knowledge and sensation of your body. Whether or not you are under supervision, it is always important to pay attention to how you feel. Anything that feels wrong or bad most likely is.

And while a class can provide supervision for you, it has a host of other requirements, such as cost, transportation, and scheduling. When you are engaging in yoga practice at home, you have the incomparable luxuries of creating your own perfect space, spending as little or as much time as you'd like practicing, and doing so whenever you desire or need to.

Here are 10 tips to help your personal yoga practice be as safe as it is beneficial:

1. The overall sensations you are trying to attain during your yoga practice are comfortable stretching and challenge, but NEVER PAIN! Anytime you feel extreme discomfort, especially in the knees or spine, do not panic, but exit the pose immediately and smoothly. Most of the discomfort you encounter in a pose can be alleviated with a few simple adjustments, and these are listed in the instructions.

2. While placing your body into new and unfamiliar positions, it is always important to breathe. In fact, the most essential aspect of any yoga pose is not the positions of the body but your awareness of the flow and quality of your own breath. Deep breathing will ground you, enhance your awareness, and leave you feeling refreshed and revitalized at the end of your session. It is often calming to extend the length of your exhalations.

3. When first learning the poses, it is a good idea to do a practice run: Read through the steps, then enter and stay in the pose for a brief time, a few breaths, before exiting and centering as you prepare to enter the pose once more. This allows you to become acquainted with the basic dynamics of the pose, as well as how to exit safely. When you have these elements down, you'll feel more free to explore the sensations of the pose itself.

4. In the beginning of your practice, allow yourself to work gradually up to greater lengths of time within each pose and for each session. Remember, the benefits of yoga are cumulative, and there is no rush. Your practice is entirely relative to your own needs and capacities.

5. A few yoga poses every day will be more beneficial than the occasional longer session. In fact, when you take note of what poses are especially relevant and provide relief to certain tight areas, you will come to crave the sensation of relaxation and expansion they provide.

6. If you are struggling with motivation, it is important to consider and identify with the long-term benefits of practice, as well as to savor the immediate pleasure of a pose accomplished and the strength and flexibility you feel afterward. Congratulate yourself.

7. Practice with another person, especially if you are concerned with balance. Have your companion spot

you on the more challenging poses. Make it a fun yoga date, ending and celebrating your practice by sharing a pot of tea or a mellow walk.

8. Always have a support, such as a chair, countertop, or even a wall nearby, so that you may reach out for support. Nearly all of these poses are adaptable, and Chapter 9, "Yoga Snacks," is especially accessible for those struggling with balance.

9. It is also useful to have several spare pillows or folded blankets on hand to support yourself in a challenging pose or relieve unnecessary pressure on any part of the body.

10. As with any new exercise regime, it is essential to check its safety and appropriateness with your doctor.

4

An Introduction to Yoga

In ancient times, yoga was often referred to as a tree, a living energy with roots in earth, trunk in middle ground, and branches reaching to the skies, uniting all three. Hatha yoga is one distinct branch, which includes the physical postures and poses pictured in this book. Other branches of yoga include Raja (meditation and spiritual practices); Karma (the path of service, giving back, volunteering); Bhakti (the path of devotion); Jnana (the path of wisdom, knowledge, and scholastic understanding); Tantra (the sacred in all we do, a reverential approach to life). Tantra has been misunderstood in the West as a sexual treatise. Tantra can be applied to sexuality, but the former definition is truly the essence of Tantra.

Sanskrit, the Indo-European language of the Vedas, India's ancient religious texts, brought forth the teachings and practice of yoga. Over time, yoga has been described as a way of uniting mind, body, and spirit—a method of discipline and practice. Yoga was passed down as an oral tradition, transmitted directly from teacher to student. The Indian sage, Patanjali, has been credited with putting this oral tradition into classical works. The Yoga Sutras are a 2,000-year-old treatise on yoga. Beginning with oral tradition, the teachings and practice of yoga are thought to be at least 5,000 years old.

The practice of yoga is accompanied by the use of calm, rhythmic breathing patterns, called *pranayama.* These practices, in a variety of forms, are also at the heart of meditation and quiet reflection. In addition, these same breathing practices can be used throughout one's day to reduce anxiety, agitation, and stress. The most universally practiced breathing technique is called "observance of the breath." Simply stated: inhale–pause–exhale.

The breath is closely tied to the mind and emotions. When our mind is agitated by anxiety, worry, or restlessness, the breath becomes rapid, shallow, and irregular. When we are calm and relaxed, the breath flows in an even, smooth, and rhythmic manner. With steady, calm breathing, as time passes, our abdominal muscles, diaphragm, and intercostal muscles will be strengthened, and eventually we make full use of our lung capacity. This slows the heartbeat, calms the nervous system, and relaxes the entire body.

It has been said by Kariba Ekken, a 17th-century mystic: "If you would foster a calm spirit, first regulate your breathing. For when that is under control, the heart will be at peace. When breathing is jagged and uneven, you will be troubled. Before attempting anything, first regulate your breathing (calm and regular) on which your temper will be softened and your spirit calmed."

Although most people cannot change their breathing habits overnight, we are designed to breathe deeply and can do this efficiently with practice over time.

PART 2

THE POSES

5

Supine Postures (Lying on Your Back)

There are always days when we just need to be restored. What's that you say? There's no 5-star resort on the next block? And the cruise ship with a spa on every deck has sailed off without you? And Jeeves, the usually wonderfully efficient butler, has failed to show up with your 5p.m. martini?

Not to worry, we have just the thing. These poses help you become empowered through relaxation.

Note: For some of the extended poses, in which you are lying for several minutes at a time, it can aid relaxation if you keep yourself comfortable beneath a warm and light blanket.

CORPSE POSE

The Corpse Pose is a classic relaxation posture that aligns the body, reduces stress and fatigue, and promotes calm.

Start from a seated position on the floor with your knees bent, feet on the floor.

Lean back onto your forearms.

Ease down gently to lie flat on your back. Slowly extend legs.

Relax your arms at your sides, comfortably away from your torso, palms up.

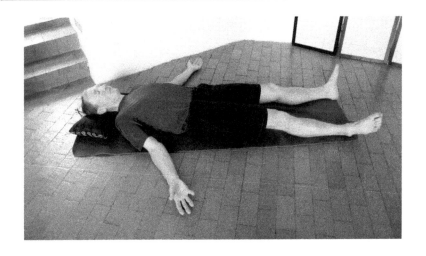

If this is not comfortable, position your arms so they are at ease.

Other modifications to make you more comfortable include:

Use a pillow or bolster to support your head.

For a more supported form of Corpse Pose, you may use several pillows or bolsters to raise the lower back and the head. This variation can open the chest, relieve congestion and counteract hunching.

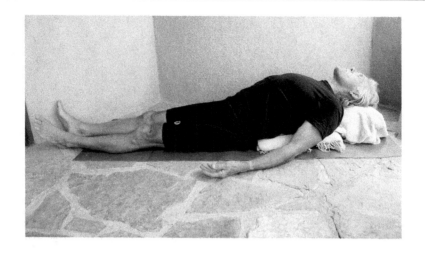

If you feel tension in your lower back, you may bend your legs, with your feet flat on the floor. Allow your knees to drop open to the sides, with bolsters or pillows supporting your thighs. If it's comfortable, allow the soles of your feet to rest against each other. Place your hands on your belly or on the floor beside you. This variation will also open your pelvis and release tension in thigh muscles.

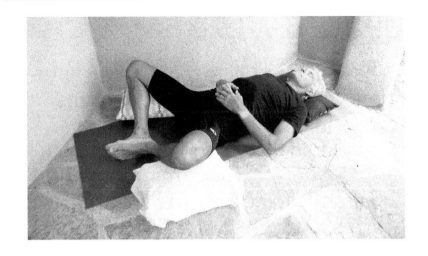

Relax.

Close your eyes and take a deep breath, allowing your attention to sweep through your body, especially through the shoulders, neck, and face, as well as the muscles around the eyes and the tongue.

Wherever you encounter tension, breathe deeply as you soothe that part into relaxation.

Remain in this pose for as long as you wish.

SUPINE TWIST

The Supine Twist facilitates range of motion in hip joints, lengthens hip flexors, and tones the abdominals.

Begin by lying on your back.

Sweep your arms up with the palms facing down so that your arms and torso create a T shape.

Bend and raise both knees to your chest.

Take a deep breath.

As you exhale, slowly lower both knees over to the left side of your body, letting the spine and the lower back twist.

Slide your knees as close to the left arm as possible. Turn your head to gaze at your right fingertips.

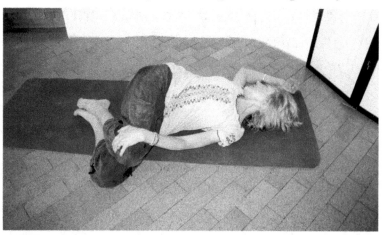

Keep your neck relaxed, and allow your shoulders to rest flat on the floor.

Close your eyes, breathe deeply, and relax into the posture. You should not make any effort in this posture, so allow gravity to pull your knees down.

Hold the pose for 6 to 10 breaths.

When you are ready to release, inhale and roll the hips back flat on the floor.

Repeat on other side.

ABDOMINAL CURL

The Abdominal Curl facilitates range of motion in the hip joints, stretches the lower back, lengthens hip flexors, tones the abdominals, and strengthens the neck. Use a pillow to support your neck if it is more comfortable.

Begin by lying on your back, with your knees bent and your feet lifted slightly off the floor.

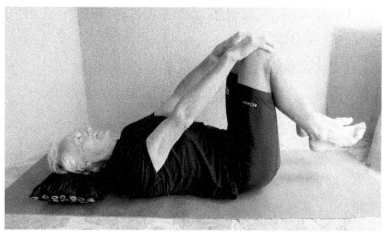

Take a deep breath.

As you exhale, raise your head, and tuck your chin down toward your chest. Hold your legs by clasping your hands at the top of the shins or underneath the knees. Bring both knees toward your chest, pressing the lower back into the floor.

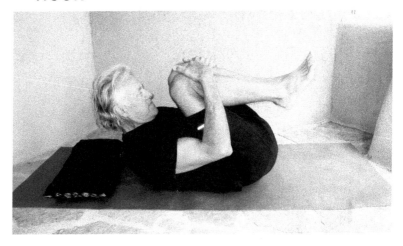

Inhale as you return to starting position.
Lengthen your exhalation with each repetition.
You may repeat this up to 10 times.

THE SINGLE LEG ABDOMINAL CURL

Begin by lying on your back, with your knees bent and your feet flat on the floor.

Take a deep breath.

As you exhale, bring your right thigh toward your chest.

Hold your leg by clasping your hands at the top part of your shin or underneath the knee.

Point your chin down toward your chest.

Straighten the left leg on the floor.

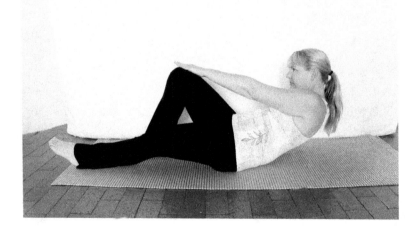

Hold for 1 breath.
Repeat with other leg.

Repeat up to 10 times.

SUPINE LEG STRETCH

The Supine Leg Stretch facilitates range of motion in hip joints and increases flexibility in the hamstrings and inner and outer thighs. Use a pillow to support your neck if it is more comfortable.

Begin by lying on your back, with arms at your sides, knees bent, feet flat on the floor.

Take a deep breath.

On the exhalation, bend your right leg, bringing it toward your chest.

As you inhale, flex your heel, straighten the knee, and raise your leg as straight as possible.

Keep your arms at your side, or you may bring your arms to lay on the floor over your head.

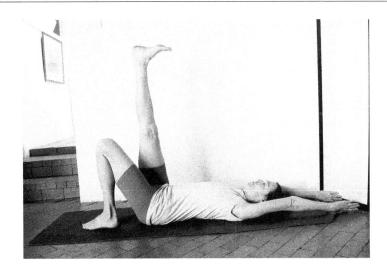

You may also hold the back of your thigh to support the pose.

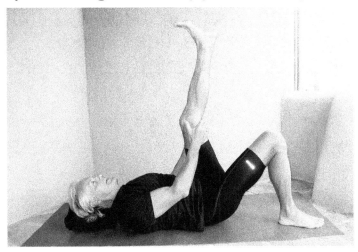

Or use a strap or belt to help increase the stretch.

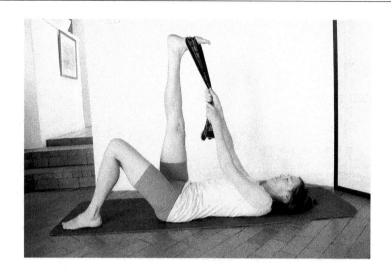

Hold, keeping your neck and shoulders relaxed.
Keeping your right leg straight, lower it to the floor.
Repeat the stretch on the left leg.

DEAD BUG POSE

The Dead Bug Pose improves circulation, relieves congestion of legs, and helps relieve lower back discomfort. Use a pillow to support your neck if it is more comfortable.

Begin by lying on your back.

Bring your knees to your chest.

Grab wherever is comfortable and possible—you may take hold of the toes, the soles of the feet, the ankles, or the back of the legs.

Slowly spread your feet apart until they are above your knees, and pull so that your knees drop toward the floor alongside your chest.

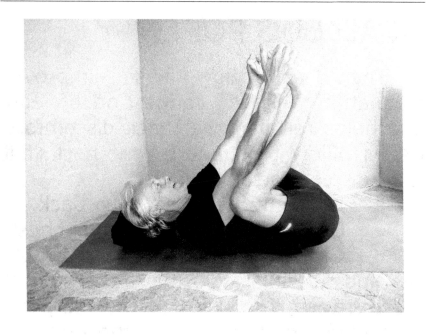

Allow your neck and shoulders
to relax while you hold the pose.

MODIFIED SHOULDER STAND

This pose improves cardiovascular health, encouraging blood flow out of the legs and into the torso. Organs and glands are gently stimulated, and tension is released from the hips.

Begin seated sideways on the floor next to a wall, with your shoulder nearly touching the wall beside you.

Breathe in deeply.

As you exhale, in one movement, while using your arms to brace your body, lower your torso and swing your legs up onto the wall so that your heels and legs are resting against it.

For a more gradual alternative to getting into the pose, you may begin the pose while lying parallel to the wall, and gradually lift your legs up the wall until your heels and the back of your legs are straight and resting against it.

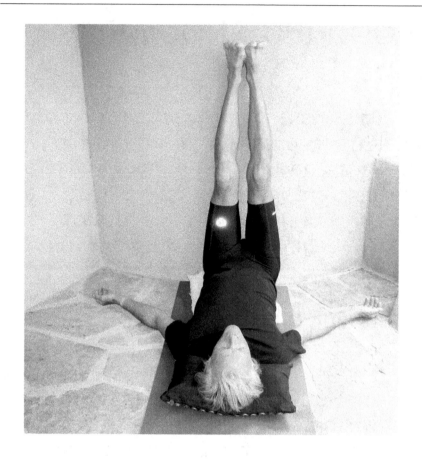

If you feel any tightness or discomfort in your lower back, push yourself away from the wall.

If the lower back discomfort remains, place a folded thick towel or pillow beneath your hips for support.

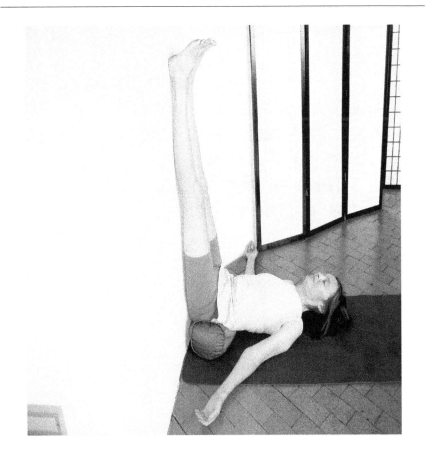

If there is discomfort in your neck, place a small pillow or folded towel beneath your neck for support.

Make sure your back is straight and your knees are not locked. Allow your neck and shoulders, arms, and hands to relax.

Breathe deeply as you hold the pose. You may stay in this pose for a few breaths or up to several minutes.

To exit the pose, simply reverse the movement by swinging or slowly easing your legs along the wall down to the floor.

Take a breath, and rest for an extra moment before rising.

BRIDGE POSE

The Bridge Pose increases flexibility in the front body and thighs while strengthening the spine. It is stimulating to the spine and body in general.

Begin by lying on the floor. If you need to protect your neck in this pose, you may place a towel or soft pillow beneath your shoulders.

With your knees bent, feet flat on the floor, bring your heels in as close as comfortable toward your sitting bones.

Breathe deeply, and as you inhale, press down into your feet and raise your hips toward the ceiling. Your weight should be resting on your feet and shoulders. The muscles through your back, buttocks, and the back of your legs should be engaged.

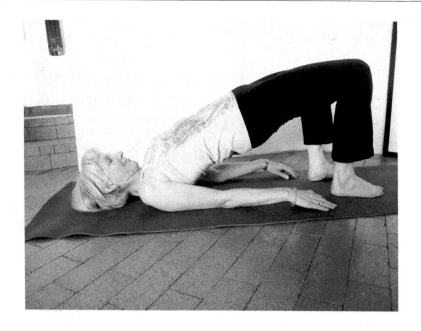

Let your arms lie along your side.

Exhale as you lower yourself and inhale as you raise yourself again. Do this 3 times before holding the pose, to gradually introduce the pose to your body.

Do a final lift, and breathe deeply as you hold the pose.

When you are ready to exit, slowly release your muscles as you lower yourself gently to the floor.

6

Prone Postures (on Knees or Belly)

Discovering that you have Parkinson's disease (PD) is devastating and scary, but it can also be an opportunity for reflection and discovery. As peace activist and Buddhist monk Thich Nhat Hanh puts it, "Life is filled with suffering, but it is also filled with many wonders, like the blue sky, the sunshine, the eyes of a baby. To suffer is not enough. We must also be in touch with the wonders of life."

These prone poses call upon the core of your body, summoning its flexibility and strength. As you go through them, make this a multidimensional practice. As you challenge your core muscles, honor the inner strength that comes forth from your being. Acknowledge your flexibility in both body and mind. As you stretch and bend your body, see how you may also turn your attention to the beautiful and encouraging aspects of life.

Note: Depending on the flexibility of your hips and knees, some of these poses may be more comfortable and appropriate for you than others. It is important that you pay attention to the sensations created by each pose. If any discomfort arises, attempt to use the supports described, or try the alternate forms of the pose, if provided. If discomfort persists, however, it is important that you do not push your body into injury. Respect and honor your capacities, and seek poses that feel both expansive and nurturing. If you have knee issues, or have recently undergone knee surgery, it is imperative that you receive your doctor's permission to engage in these poses.

You may benefit from supports for the following poses. If your hips are tight or you have difficulty keeping your back straight in these poses, raising your hips to be level or above your knees may grant relief. To do this, you may use a folded towel or blanket as support. Begin seated on the blanket, then scoot gently off until you are barely perched upon it, and it is only lifting your hips and tailbone a few inches off the floor.

Also, if you are experiencing tightness in your groin, you may place the supports of folded blankets beneath your knees. After holding the pose, you may find that after removing the supports, your muscles may have relaxed, allowing you to stretch more deeply into the pose.

CAT POSE

The Cat Pose creates flexibility in the pelvis and spine and builds strength in the arms.

Begin on your hands and knees, with wrists beneath the shoulders and knees below the hips.

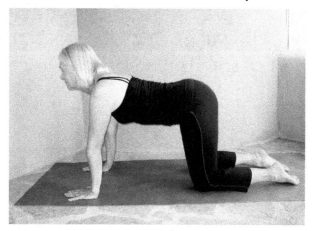

Hold your spine in a neutral position, neither tense nor sagging toward the floor, but in a straight strong line, with your neck held as an extension of that line.

Take a deep breath.

As you exhale, gradually contract your abdominal muscles up toward your spine, at the same time tilting your pelvis and contracting your buttocks so that your tailbone points down toward the floor.

Pressing your hands firmly into the floor, push up through your shoulders, rounding your back toward the ceiling. Allow your head to curl under, so that you are looking at the floor between your knees.

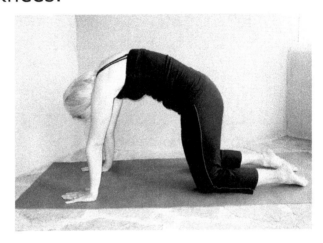

Hold this pose for several breaths.

Then, shift into the next part of the pose.

As you inhale, release the tension in your buttocks and reverse the tilt of your pelvis. Allow your abdomen to lower toward the floor as you reverse the arch of your back and raise your head to gaze up at the ceiling.

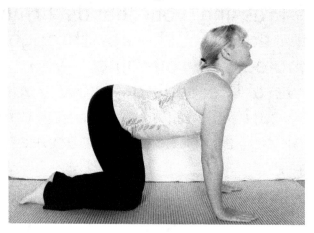

Do not over bend your spine into discomfort, but keep it in a strong, smooth arch.

Go back and forth between the two positions, always shifting the pelvis first, then allowing that motion to move like a wave up through your spine, with your neck completing the motion. Exhale as you arch your back up toward the ceiling, and inhale as you drop your abdomen towards the floor.

Pay attention to the flow and strength of the wave motion going through your spine.

CHILD'S POSE

The Child's Pose brings circulation to the lower back and abdominals, stimulates the organs of the pelvic region, relieves lower back tension, and stretches hips, thighs, and ankles.

Begin on your hands and knees.

Move your hips toward your heels, your chest and torso to your thighs, and your forehead to the floor. If you like, you may place a pillow on the floor before you and rest your forehead on that.

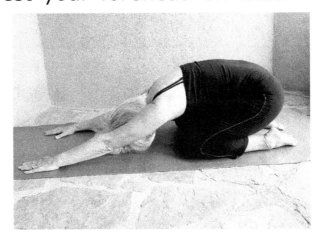

If this is uncomfortable, you may place a pillow between your torso and thighs, another behind your knees, a third under your ankles, and one for your head to rest on.

The entire body folds into a fetal position.

For a longer stay, bring your arms to rest alongside your body, palms up.

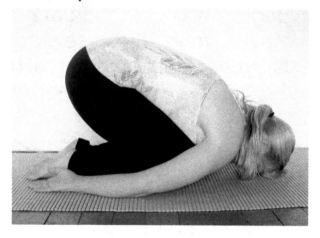

Hold for 3 to 5 breaths or longer if desired.

COBRA POSE

The Cobra Pose strengthens the back muscles, arms, and abdominals, opens the chest, and improves posture.

Begin this pose lying face down on the floor with your palms flat on the floor beneath your shoulders and the tops of your feet flat on the floor.

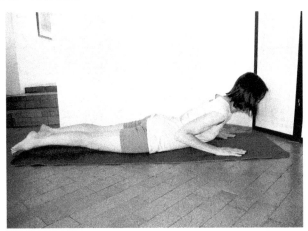

Take a deep breath.

As you inhale, slowly straighten your elbows, bringing your chest up and arching your back, keeping your spine extended. Allow your thighs to press down into the floor and your chest to point upward and outward.

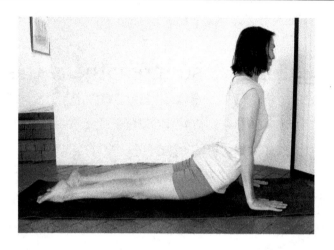

Do not push the stretch or over-tense any of your muscles, but allow yourself to breathe easily as you hold the pose.

Hold pose for 3 to 5 breaths.

DIAGONAL STRETCH POSE

The Diagonal Stretch Pose is a great back strengthener that stretches diagonally across the spine (first one way and then the other), allowing the back muscles to let go of tension.

Begin this pose lying on your stomach with the tops of your feet flat on the floor and your chin resting on the floor.

Bend one leg up and reach back with the arm from the same side of your body to grab your foot or ankle, wherever it is most comfortable.

While maintaining this hold, exhale and reach your other arm forward, pointing it.

Point your free foot, and feel the energy coursing through the line from your foot to your hand.

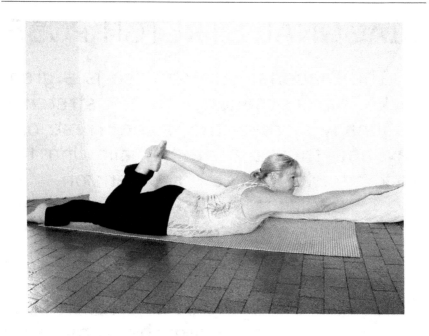

Hold this pose for 15 seconds or as long as comfortable.

Exhale and release the pose, then repeat on the other side.

HALF-CIRCLE POSE

The Half-Circle Pose is side stretch that opens the belly and chest, stretching and strengthening the arms, shoulders, chest, and abdomen.

Begin this pose kneeling, with your knees hip width apart.

Step your left leg sideways, placing your left foot flat on the floor, pointed forward.

Slowly lower your right hand to rest on the floor directly beneath your right shoulder.

Inhale as you raise your left hand over your head.

As you exhale, press your hips forward, arch your back, and turn your head to gaze up at your hand.

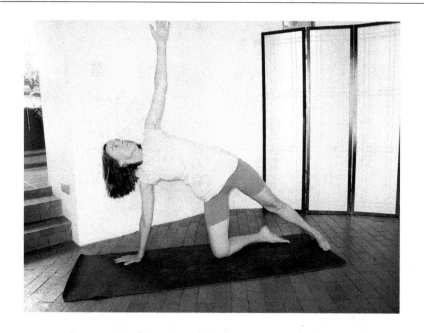

The right side of your body will now be making a half-circle shape.

Hold this pose for 3 to 8 breaths before releasing the pose and repeating on the other side.

7

Seated Poses

Seated postures focus on the torso and hips. Practicing these poses will ground and calm you. As you go through them, pay attention to what allows the muscles of your back to relax. Doing a few of these poses before bedtime may release tension and ensure a better night's sleep. Enjoy the tranquility you'll discover in these poses.

The Seated Poses remind me that sitting can change the way you see the world. Recently I was in Avignon, France, standing in a long line at a pharmacy. Out of the blue, a gallant (and handsome) gentleman who worked there brought me a chair.

Later on that same trip, I was in Paris, stumbling into a bistro when the owner came dashing over to help me get seated at a nearby table. The best part is that he removed a "Reserved" sign from this table and put it elsewhere. It turns out that this lovely man was also the chef, and after an amazing dinner, he shared with me some of his grandmother's recipes.

So, seat yourself, and look for the kindness of strangers. Let these memories and positive feelings follow you into your yoga practice.

EASY POSE

This is a calming pose in preparation for relaxation and meditation.

Begin this pose seated on the floor.

If your hips are tight, you may use a folded towel or blanket as support. To set up this support, begin seated on the blanket, then scoot gently off until you are barely perched upon it, and it is only lifting your hips and tailbone a few inches off the floor.

Fold your legs in a comfortable cross-legged position.

Pull one heel in toward your groin. Depending on comfort, you may lay the other heel on top of the opposite leg, or allow it to rest on the floor before you.

Place your hands on your thighs or feet.

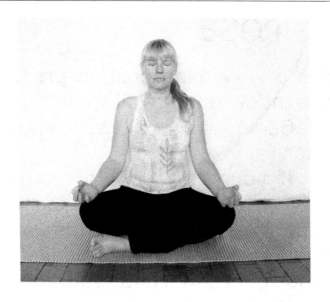

As you breathe deeply, allow your shoulders to relax and your shoulder blades to slide down your back.

Press the crown of your head away from the shoulders, creating stretch and elongation in your spine.

You may hold this pose as long as you are comfortable.

Hold the pose, breathe deeply, then release, and repeat with the opposite leg on top.

SEATED TWIST POSE

The Seated Twist Pose strengthens muscles of the front and torso and promotes flexibility in hip joints in the lower back.

You may practice this pose seated on the floor or on a chair, according to your capacity and comfort.

Seated Twist, Floor Version

Begin seated on the floor, with your knees bent and your feet flat on the floor before you.

Lower your left leg to the floor, extending straight in front of you.

Cross your right leg over your left leg so that your right foot rests flat on the floor.

Bring your left elbow across your right knee, and use it to gently push against the outside of your knee, creating a twist through your torso.

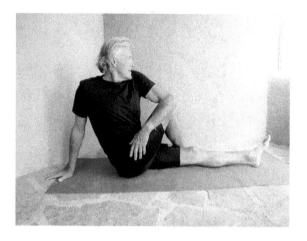

You may keep your left arm up, or relax it to lie down along your right outer thigh.

Fold your right hand over your left, or lay your hand on the floor behind you, and use it to brace your body. Keep a slight bend in your elbow so that it does not lock.

Look behind you, and as you inhale, elongate your spine, stretching it up toward the ceiling. As you exhale, press your left elbow against your right knee, easing yourself into a deeper twist.

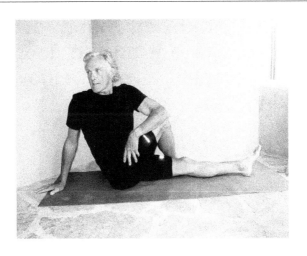

Hold this pose for several breaths before you release and come to center. Extend both your legs to lie straight on the floor before you and take a few deep breaths before you repeat on the opposite side.

Keep your right leg lying flat on the floor. Bend your left knee as you raise and cross your left leg over your right, so that your left foot rests flat on the floor.

Bring your right elbow across the outside of the left knee, pressing against it to deepen the twist through your spine.

Keep your right arm up or relax it down your left thigh.

Fold your left hand over your right, or place it on the floor behind you, keeping your elbow from locking.

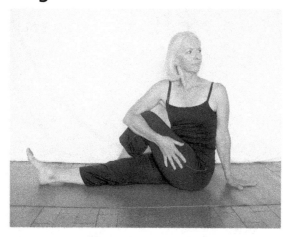

Look behind you. As you inhale, extend your spine. As you exhale, press deeper into the pose. Hold for several breaths before you release the pose and come back to center.

FORWARD BEND POSE

The Forward Bend Pose stretches legs and hamstrings, opens hips, tones and stimulates the internal organs, strengthens and elongates the spine.

Begin seated on the floor with your legs stretched out in front of you. Sit with your spine as long and tall as possible. Allow your knees to bend slightly, or place a pillow or folded blanket beneath your knees.

Breathe deeply, lifting your chest and raising your hands above your head.

Hinge at your hips, and bend your torso forward, keeping your back long and straight.

Lower yourself as far as you can without compromising the straightness and length of your back.

Lower your hands to rest on your feet or legs.

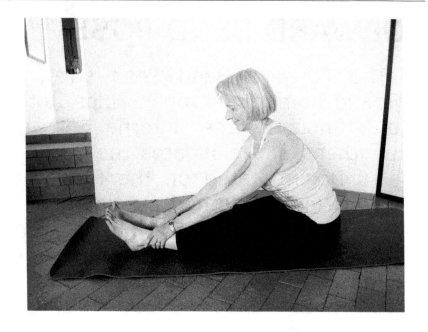

Hold the pose for 3 to 5 breaths, remembering to breathe deeply.

On an inhalation, raise your body upright, reaching your arms above your head once more, and on an exhalation, bring them back down in prayer position before your heart.

MODIFIED FORWARD BEND POSE

The Modified Forward Bend Pose stretches inner thighs and hamstrings, opens hips, tones and stimulates internal organs, strengthens and elongates the spine.

Begin seated on the floor with your legs stretched out in front of you. Sit with your spine as long and tall as possible.

Allowing your torso to lean back slightly, spread your legs apart until you feel a good stretch.

If you feel any pain in your inner thighs or knees, bring your legs in closer together.

If your hamstrings are tight, you can allow your knees to bend slightly, or even place a pillow or folded blanket beneath your knees. If you are having trouble sitting up straight, you may sit on a folded blanket or pillow.

Flex your feet so your toes are pointing toward the sky.

Place your hands on the floor between your legs.

Take a deep breath, and as you exhale, slowly walk the hands forward, hinging at the hips and keeping the spine long.

Lower yourself until you feel a good stretch in your inner thighs and along the backs of your legs. Go only as far as you can while keeping your spine straight.

Depending on how close to the floor you can lower your torso, place your forearms on the floor with hands clasped, or stretch your arms out straight in front of you with your hands flat on the floor.

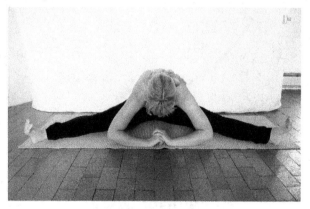

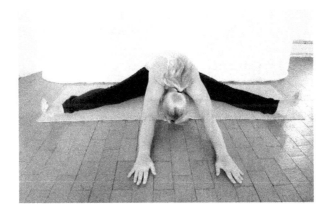

At the beginning, you may not be able to lean forward very much. This is fine. Simply stay in the pose with your legs wide, breathing deeply. With repeated practice, you will gain flexibility and be able to lean further forward.

Hold this pose for 3 to 5 breaths. On your exhalations, see if you can relax deeper into the stretch.

To exit the pose, walk your hands back up until your torso is upright. Take a breath before slowly bringing your legs back together in front of you.

BUTTERFLY POSE

The Butterfly Pose helps tendons running into the groin remain limber and elastic and promotes mobility and limberness of the hips and lower back.

Begin seated on the floor with your legs stretched out in front of you. If you find that your back starts to hunch, sit upon a firm pillow or folded blanket, so that your knees are below your hips.

Bend your legs and bring the soles of your feet together. Place your hands over your feet to keep them in place.

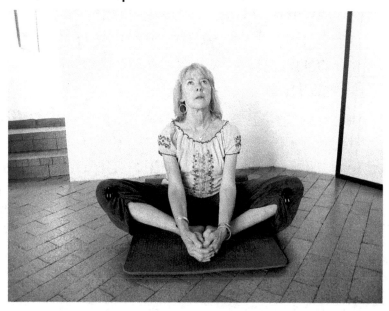

You may pull your feet closer into the body to intensify the stretch in your hamstrings.

If you are still having trouble with keeping a straight back, you may place your hands on the floor behind you to support your posture.

Breathe deeply as you allow your groin muscles to relax in the pose. They will gradually release, letting your legs naturally ease down closer to the floor.

To intensify the stretch, you may bend forward. Do not bend your spine, but hinge at the hips, dropping your belly to the floor as you keep your spine long and straight. You may place your hands flat on the floor before you or clasp them over your feet.

Hold for 3 to 5 breaths. If you like, you may hold this pose for a longer period as well.

To exit the pose, come upright, release your hold on your feet, stretch your legs out before you, and take a deep breath before continuing to the next pose.

8

Standing Postures

Standing poses challenge and encourage good posture and stamina. Your awareness of the balance within your body will be strengthened and enhanced through these poses. To become more aware of your posture, realize your body expands in two directions: Let yourself connect to the earth through a solid stance, as you are also drawn up toward the sky through a lifted head and straight spine.

MOUNTAIN POSE

This pose is the basis of all standing poses. It's a good pose for encouraging good posture and balance and helps you to establish a feeling of stability. It also promotes inner calm.

Begin by standing with your feet parallel to each other, hip width apart.

Your feet should be directly below your knees, and your knees should be directly below your hips, so that there is a strong line of support through your lower limbs.

Pay attention to the sensation of your feet against the floor. Spread your toes, and imagine that each of your feet has four corners that are resting solidly on the ground, making your feet wide and stable bases for the rest of your body.

As you breathe, check to make sure your weight is distributed evenly. If you notice that you are leaning more on one foot or another, or forward or backward, gently correct your stance.

Place your hands together in a prayer position in front of your heart, or let them relax at your sides.

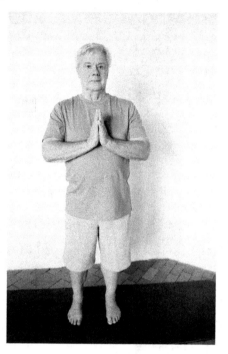

Keep your gaze at eye level on a point directly in front of you.

Take a deep breath, letting your chest lift up as it expands with your breath, extending your spine, so you stand taller, allowing your shoulders to relax and roll back as your spine lengthens.

Lift your kneecaps up by contracting the front of your thigh. Do not let your knees lock.

Engage the muscles in back of your thighs and buttocks.

Let your mind still, and feel in the pose the solidity and calmness of a mountain.

LATERAL NECK STRETCH

The Lateral Neck Stretch keeps the neck muscles limber and flexible.

Begin in Mountain Pose, with the chin tucked in.

Slowly drop your ear down toward your shoulder until you are at full stretch. Hold the pose for five breaths, allowing yourself to relax deeper into the pose with each exhalation.

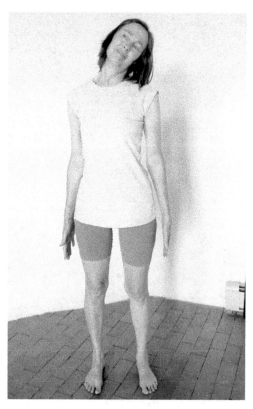

Then lift your head slowly back to center, take a breath, and repeat on the other side.

STANDING TREE POSE

The Standing Tree Pose develops balance, concentration, and calm. It promotes hip flexibility and gives a sense of confidence and character to one's physical presence.

This pose may be performed in several different variations. The variations are listed from least to most challenging. Choose the form that is best for you.

For extra support and balance, use a chair or wall for support.

The most stable form of Tree Pose:

Begin in Mountain Pose.

Take a deep breath, and as you exhale, raise your hands straight up, keeping your fingers pointed up toward the sky.

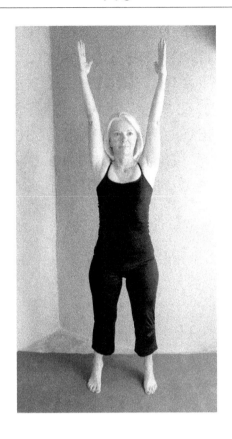

While keeping your hands raised, breathe again, allowing your shoulders and neck muscles to relax.

Hold this pose for 5 breaths before slowly lowering the arms and returning to Mountain Pose.

A more challenging form of Tree Pose:

Begin in Mountain Pose.

If you have the support of a chair or a wall at your side, shift your weight to the foot farthest away from the support.

Lift the foot closest to the support, and bring it in toward the other leg. Rest your sole against the inner ankle of the standing leg, with the toes pointing down.

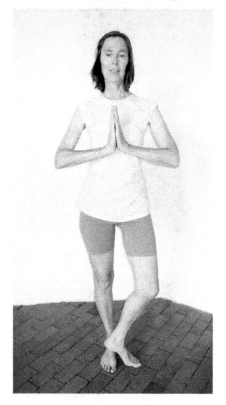

Alternatively, you may raise your foot higher, and rest it anywhere along the inside of your standing leg, always with the toes pointing down. The higher you raise your foot, the more the pose will challenge your balance.

For the full extent of the pose, place the sole of the foot at the very top of the inner thigh on the standing leg. You may use your hands to help yourself position your foot if you raise it this high.

Do not allow your bent leg to come forward—keep it out to the side, creating a stretch through your pelvis.

When you have positioned your foot, you may either bring your hands together before your heart, or, for even more of a balance challenge, raise them straight up above your head. If you are using a support, lean with one arm and allow the other to rest at your side.

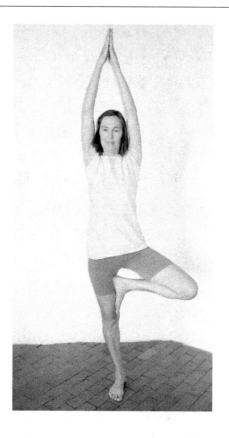

To help with balance, keep your gaze fixed on an object at eye level directly in front of you.

Keeping your spine straight and your shoulders relaxed, hold for 5 breaths before slowly coming out of the pose.

Center yourself in Mountain Pose for one breath, then turn to reverse the orientation of your support before you repeat on the other side.

HALF-SQUAT POSE

The Half-Squat Pose increases flexibility in lower back, hips, and calves. It strengthens buttocks and hamstrings and is helpful for digestion and elimination.

Begin in Mountain Pose.

Bend your knees, and let your torso tilt diagonally forward, as if you are going to sit on a chair.

Place your hands on your legs, and actively press your heels into the floor. This should relieve tension in your lower back and hips.

Keep your back long, without hunching or arching. Tuck your tailbone slightly so that it is pointed straight down at the ground.

Bring your arms up. If your shoulders are flexible, you may raise your arms above your head, setting them to continue on the same diagonal angle as your torso. However, if you find that this makes you hunch your back, you may set your arms at a lower angle, or place them together in a prayer position in front of your heart.

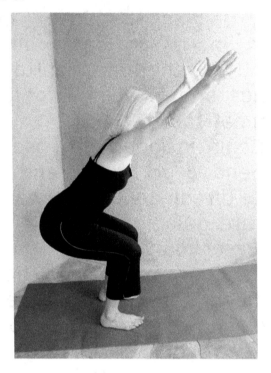

Hold for a few breaths before standing to release the pose.

TRIANGLE POSE

The Triangle Pose strengthens legs and encourages flexibility in the hips. It stretches and strengthens the musculature of the torso.

Begin by standing with feet 3 to 4 feet apart.

Keeping your right foot still and pointed forward, swivel on the heel of your left foot until your toes are pointing out and to the left, and your left foot is at a perpendicular angle to your right.

Make sure your heels are aligned and your weight is distributed evenly over both your feet.

Take a deep breath and raise your arms up to a T position. Keep your shoulders relaxed.

Slowly lean laterally to your left, gradually shifting your weight to rest a bit more on the left foot.

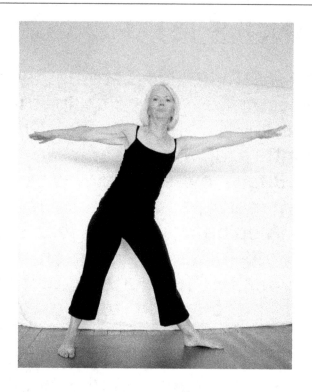

On exhalation, reach your left hand out and over, then down to your left leg or foot as you reach the full extension of the pose.

You may rest your left hand on your leg, ankle, chair seat or other support.

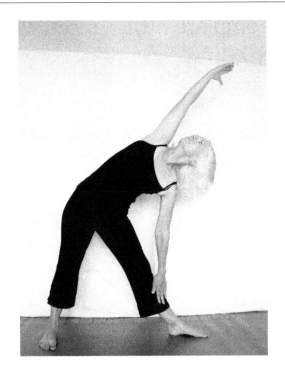

By rotating your torso right, you can keep both sides feeling equally extended.

Keep the right foot strongly rooted to the floor. Stay for 3 to 5 breaths.

On inhalation, look up toward the extended right hand, on exhalation, look down to the left foot.

Return to upright on the last inhalation.

Center yourself, arms in a T position, before shifting your feet to complete this stretch on the other side.

MOON SALUTE

The Moon Salute promotes balance, calm, and stamina.

Begin in Mountain Pose.

Clasp your hands lightly, and take a deep breath in as you raise them above your head.

As you exhale, tilt your arms and your torso laterally to one side, creating a shape reminiscent of a crescent moon. Make sure that you do not hunch, but keep your shoulders back, and lengthen through your arms as you push through your feet. You should feel a stretch along the side of your body.

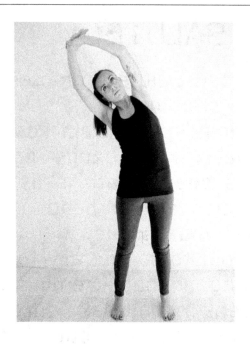

Come back to center, take a breath as you center, and then repeat the crescent on the other side.

Release your hands, and return to Mountain Pose. Once you have centered, take a deep breath.

As you exhale, step one foot out to the side, so your feet are double hip-width apart.

Bend your knees and lower your sitting bones to come down into a squat.

Keep your spine strong and long as you hold your head up straight.

Keep your elbows bent and your arms raised with your hands held at face height, fingers pointed toward the sky.

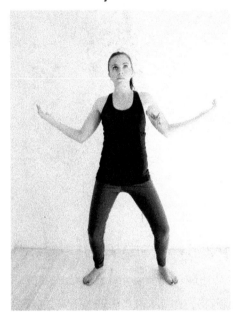

You may place a hand on a wall or chair back for added stability.

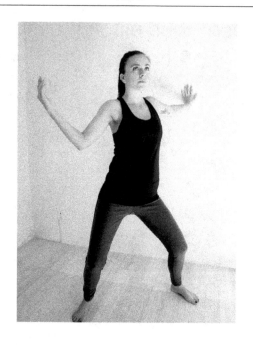

Hold for several breaths before releasing.

HIP ROTATIONS

Hip Rotations keep the mid-section of the body loose and limber. They relieve tension in the lower back.

Stand with your hands on your waist, your feet about shoulder width apart.

Shift your weight to one hip, letting your torso tilt away as you rotate your hips first in one direction several times and then in the other direction.

Make your rotations continuous and smooth.

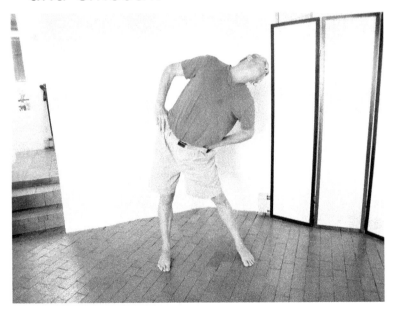

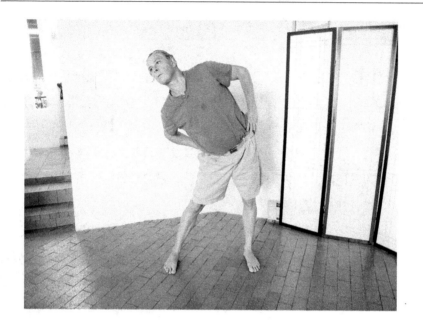

WARRIOR POSE

The Warrior Pose stretches and strengthens legs, hips, shoulders, arms, and chest. It promotes confidence and courage.

Begin by standing with feet 3 to 4 feet apart.

Raise your arms to form a T position, palms facing down.

Turn your head to the left, looking out over your hand.

Turn your left foot 90 degrees to the left, so that your toes are pointing in the same direction as you are facing.

Bend your left knee until it lines up directly over your left ankle.

Press your right heel firmly into the floor, which will help your right leg remain straight.

Keeping your arms extended, make sure that your torso is centered, with your shoulders directly above your pelvis. Keep your spine long, with your chest raised and open and your abdomen engaged.

Keep your arms extended strongly out at shoulder height. Gaze beyond the outstretched left hand.

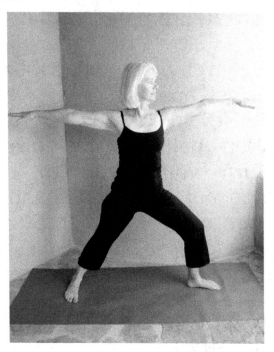

To exit pose, straighten your left leg, come to center, take a breath, and then repeat the pose on the other side.

CLASSIC FORWARD BEND

The Classic Forward Bend preserves mobility of hip joints, elongates and stretches the lower back, and massages organs.

Begin in Mountain Pose.

Breathe deeply, and on an exhalation, bend slowly forward, hinging at the waist. Keep your spine long and straight. You may bend your knees slightly. Drop your hands down to the floor, to your feet, or to wherever on your legs you can comfortably rest them.

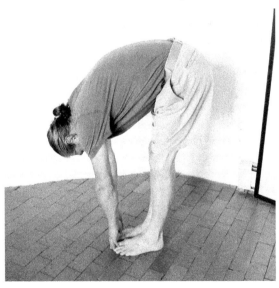

With each breath, try to release any tension in the hips and lower back, and ease deeper into the stretch.

Hold for 10 breaths and come slowly back up to Mountain Pose.

SUPPORTED STANDING FORWARD BEND

This pose stretches the back and hamstrings and encourages the ability to hinge at the hips. It provides gentle traction, encouraging straightness and counteracting compression of the spine. It strengthens the back and reminds the spine of correct straight posture.

Place hands on a stable table, chair, or countertop.

Step back, folding at the hips, until the arms and spine are extended, and your upper torso is parallel to the floor.

Tuck your chin.

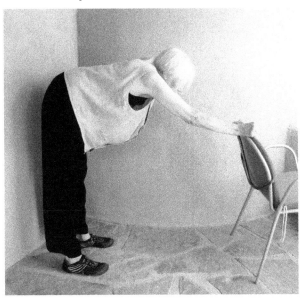

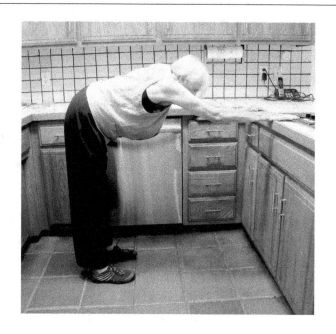

Focus on spinal extension.
Stay in position for 3 to 5 breaths.

MODIFIED FORWARD BEND (HALF BEND)

These variations allow you to perform the Forward Bend with a greater amount of stability.

Variation 1:

Begin in Mountain Pose.

Fold your arms over your chest, and bend your torso forward, hinging at the hips and keeping your spine long and straight.

Bend far enough that you feel a stretch through your hamstrings and back, while keeping them straight.

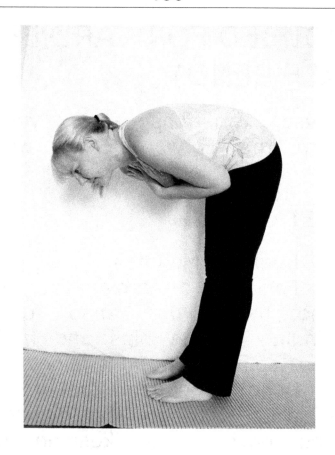

If your hamstrings are very tight, this will stretch them without overtaxing. If you are concerned about your stability, you may perform this pose above a chair.

Variation 2:

Begin in Mountain Pose.
Taking a deep breath, inhale, and sweep your arms up gracefully over your head.

Keeping your arms extended, lean your torso forward until it is nearly parallel with the floor.

Look over your hands as if you are Superman. If there is too much tension in your hamstrings, allow your knees to bend.

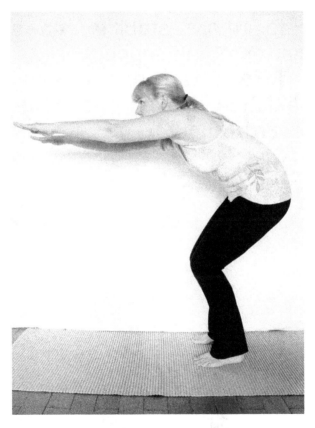

Take a deep breath, and raise your torso upright, allowing your arms to sweep back gracefully to your sides on an exhalation.

MODIFIED FORWARD BEND, WITH BENT LEG

This pose also strengthens thigh muscles.

Begin in Mountain Pose.

Place your hands on your hips, or for more stability, on a chair back or other support.

Take a deep breath, and on the exhalation, take one large step forward, about 2 feet.

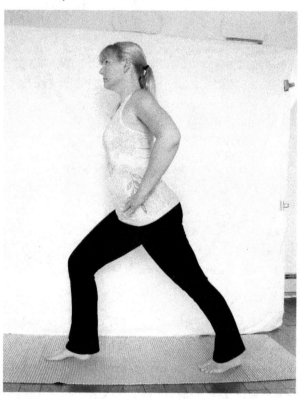

After another breath, lower your torso, hinging at the waist. Keep your spine straight.

Reach down with both hands, placing your fingertips on the floor on either side of your foremost foot. If you cannot reach the floor, you may rest them on your leg, or keep hold of a support.

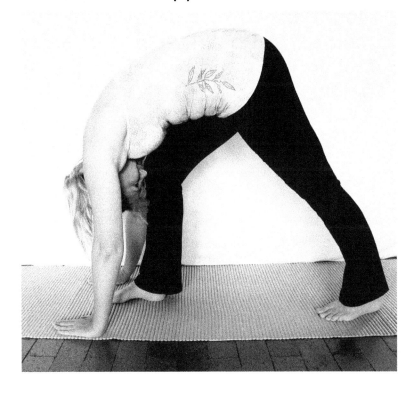

Hold for 3 to 5 breaths.

If you would like to deepen the pose, you may place your palms on the floor and bring your forehead in toward your shin.

When you are ready to release the pose, lift your head, bring your hands to your hips.

Keeping spine straight, hinge at the hips as you bring your torso back to an upright position.

Bring your feet back together in Mountain Pose and breathe for a moment before stepping the other foot forward and repeating the pose on the other side.

FORWARD BEND TWIST

The Forward Bend Twist strengthens legs and back muscles, tones the waist, and opens hips and shoulders.

Begin in Mountain Pose.

Breathe deeply, and on an exhalation, bend slowly forward, hinging at the waist. Keep your spine long and straight. You may bend your knees slightly.

Drop your hands down to the floor, to your feet, or to wherever on your legs you can comfortably rest them.

With each breath, try to release any tension in the hips and lower back, and ease deeper into the stretch.

Take your left hand to the outer right shin or to the right foot. Use that contact to push against as you twist your belly and spine.

You may place your right hand on your hip, or raise it above your head.

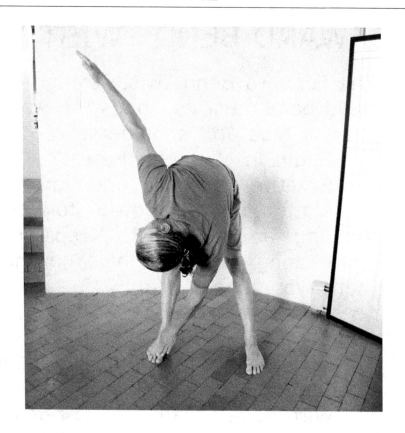

Turn your head to gaze up at your raised hand. Breathe deeply.

Come back to center, then repeat on the other side.

To exit, come back to a centered forward bend. Take your hands to your hips, inhale, and slowly come back to standing position.

STANDING TWIST

The Standing Twist is calming and releases tension throughout the back. It stimulates the internal organs, improving digestion and elimination.

Stand with a countertop on your right side.

Step your left foot forward about 2 feet.

With arms extended, place your right hand on the countertop in front, and your left hand on the countertop behind you.

Turn your head to gaze over your left shoulder.

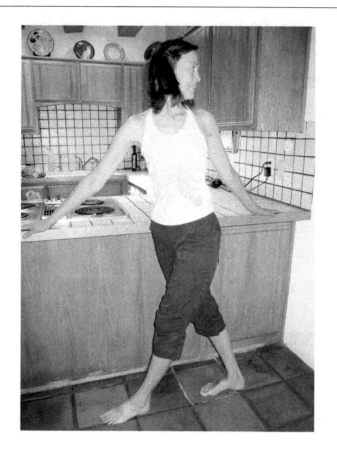

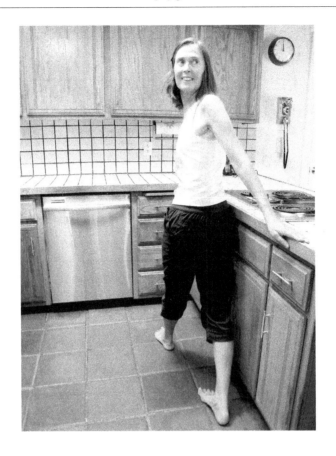

Stand tall, and enjoy this twist for a few breaths.

Release the pose and come to center before turning around and repeating the pose on the other side.

Stand with the countertop on your left side.

Step your right foot forward about 2 feet.

Place your left hand on the countertop in front of you, and your right hand on the countertop behind you.

Let your head turn to gaze over your right shoulder.

Stand tall and breathe deep as you hold the pose.

Release the pose, bringing legs, arms and face back into Mountain Pose.

FORWARD DIVE

The Forward Dive creates stimulation and flexibility for the back, legs, and shoulders. It improves balance and coordination.

Begin in Mountain Pose with your hands on your hips.

Take a deep breath. As you exhale, bend forward, hinging at the hips, until your torso is parallel with the floor.

Keep your back straight. If it is difficult to straighten your back, bend your knees slightly.

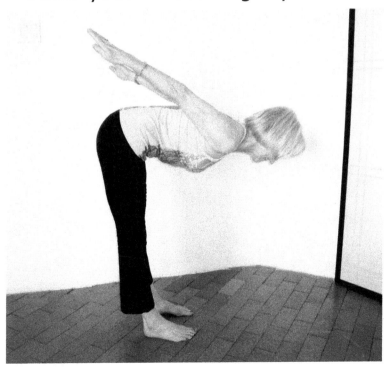

Keep your hands on your hips, or place them down on the floor, chair seat or other support placed before you. For a greater stretch through the chest and shoulders, you may lift your straight arms behind you, as pictured.

Hold the pose for several breaths. On your inhalations, try to stretch your spine, increasing the distance between your head and hips. On your exhalations, allow yourself to sink deeper into the pose.

To exit the pose, place your hands on your hips and slightly bend your knees. Engage your abdominal muscles, take a deep breath, and as you inhale, bring your torso upright.

BACKWARD BEND POSE

The Backward Bend Pose releases muscle tension in mid-lower back and stretches arms, shoulders, and neck.

To ensure the safety of this pose, your legs must be strongly engaged.

Begin in Mountain Pose, making sure that your toes are spread and your feet are wide and stable bases for your legs.

Flex your quadriceps, and tilt your pelvis forward, as if in cat pose. Keep your buttocks soft.

Breathe deeply, and as you exhale, gracefully sweep your arms up and over your head.

Allow yourself to lean back as you continue the exhalation. Feel your abdomen engage to support your spine.

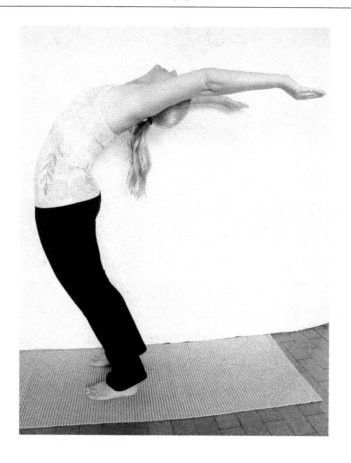

Hold the pose for 3 to 5 breaths before letting your arms sweep back down to your sides and coming upright.

Should you feel any sharp pain or discomfort during the pose, immediately and smoothly exit the pose.

STANDING SHOULDER SQUEEZE

These two variations of the Standing Shoulder Squeeze release tension from the shoulders and upper back.

Variation 1:

Begin in Mountain Pose.

Bending your knees slightly, clasp your hands loosely behind you.

Roll your upper arms out and back, which will widen and lift your chest.

Keeping your arms straight and your hands clasped, gently lift your hands until you feel a pleasant stretch through your upper arms, shoulders and upper back.

Hold for 2 breaths, allowing each breath to lift and expand the ribcage.

Release and gently bring the hands back to your sides.

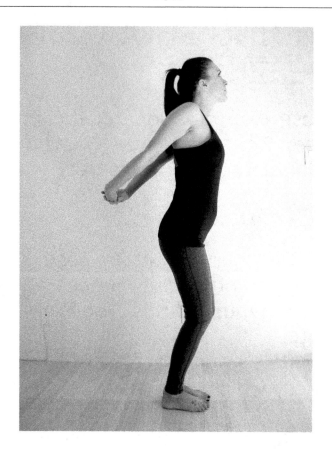

Variation 2:

Begin in Mountain Pose.

Clasp your hands loosely in front of you.

Take a deep breath. On the exhalation, lift your arms up over your head. While you are lifting your arms, keep your hands clasped, shifting your palms out and up so that when your hands are fully extended, your palms are facing the sky.

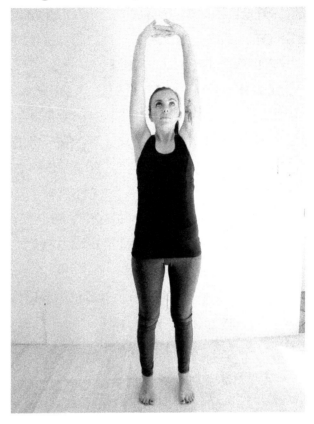

Keep your spine long and your neck and shoulders relaxed as you hold the pose.

Hold for 2 breaths before releasing your hands and letting them fall gracefully back to your sides.

LATERAL SIDE BEND

The Lateral Side Bend stretches side muscles of the back and buttocks and keeps arm and shoulder area limber.

Begin in Mountain Pose.

You have several options for hand position in this pose. You may place your hands in prayer position before your heart; then, keeping them joined, raise them above your head. Or you may clasp them together lightly.

Inhale and raise your arms over your head with your hands in the position of your choice.

Exhale and bend your body laterally to your left, stretching through your entire right side.

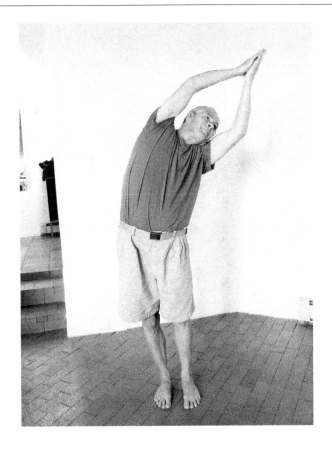

Hold for 3 to 5 breaths before returning upright, taking a breath to center, then repeat on the other side.

If you are concerned about stability, you can let the arm on the stretching side of the body continue the arc of the stretch, while the other hand braces against the adjacent outer thigh.

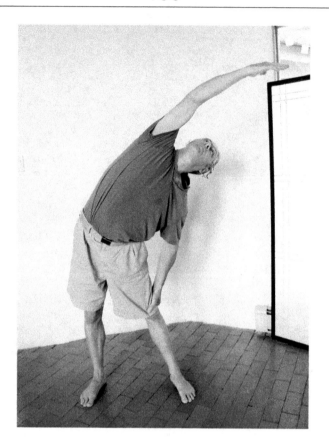

9

Yoga Snacks: Approachable Postures to Begin Your Day or When You Have Limited Time or Energy

Connie Fisher, my Viniyoga-trained yoga teacher, first introduced me to yoga snacks: approachable postures that you can do when you're crunched for time and only have a moment to spare, or you simply feel you cannot do more than a few minutes of yoga. The first 8 poses of this chapter can be done before you even get out of bed in the morning. You'll find that starting your day with these will bring warmth and flexibility to stiff, painful muscles. As you know all too well, getting out of bed may be the hardest thing you do all day.

CORPSE POSE

The Corpse Pose counteracts stress and calms the body and mind. This pose engages the parasympathetic nervous system and rejuvenates the body. It is a restorative pose.

Start from a seated position on the floor with your knees bent, feet on the floor.

Lean back onto your forearms.

Ease down gently to lie flat on your back. Slowly extend your legs.

Relax your arms at your sides, comfortably away from your torso, palms up.

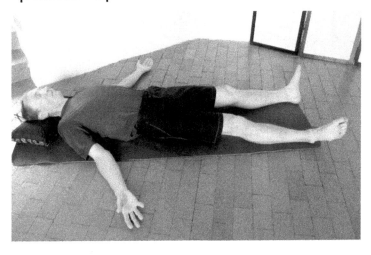

If this is not comfortable, position your arms so they are at ease. You may bend your legs, place your hands on your belly or chest, and use a pillow for your head. You may also place a light blanket over yourself to stay warm.

Relax.

Close your eyes, and take a deep breath, allowing your attention to sweep through your body, especially through the shoulders, neck, and face as well as the muscles around the eyes and the tongue.

Wherever you encounter tension, breathe deeply as you soothe that part into relaxation.

Remain in this pose for as long as you wish.

CHAIR-ASSISTED CORPSE POSE

This variation of Corpse Pose takes pressure off of the pelvis and hamstrings and allows release in the hips and lower back.

Lie on your back.

Place your lower legs comfortably on the seat of a chair.

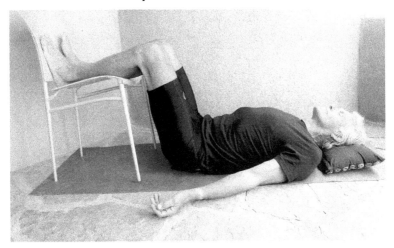

Relax.

You may remain in this pose for 5 to 10 minutes.

You may use a pillow or folded blanket beneath your head, and one beneath your knees for support. Also, since this pose is held for a

longer time, covering yourself with
a blanket will keep you warm.

KNEE HUG

The Knee Hug relaxes and stretches the back and aids in digestion and elimination.

Lie on your back with your hands on bent knees.

On exhalation, bring your knees toward your chest.

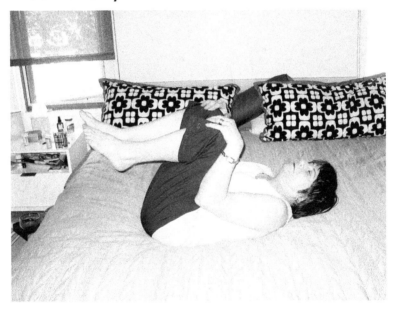

As you inhale, keep your hands on your knees. You may hold this as a still pose or introduce some movements for different effects. To massage the muscles in your back, you can rock left to right. To help the muscles in your lower back relax, you can open and close your legs like a clam.

Hold the pose or repeat the movement of your choice until your back is relaxed.

LYING TWIST

The Lying Twist stretches and relaxes the spine and releases tension throughout the back. It stimulates the internal organs, improving digestion and elimination. Twists rotate vertebrae; this compression and stretching action increases spinal strength and flexibility.

Lie on your back.

Bend your knees, place the soles of your feet on the floor, and your arms extended out to the side, palms down.

On exhalation, drop your knees to the right side, turning your head left.

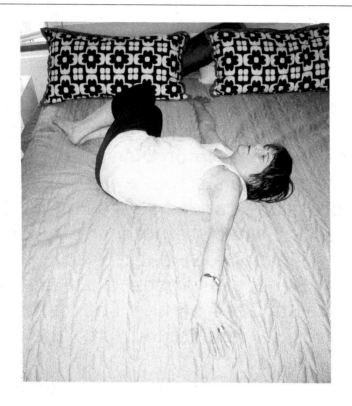

Stay 5 to 10 breaths.

Return to center on an inhalation, and repeat on the other side.

CAT POSE

This pose is excellent for releasing stress. It stretches all the way up the back through the neck and massages the internal organs.

Start on all fours, knees under hips, hands and elbows under shoulders, gazing at the floor.

Take a deep breath.

On the exhalation, round your back toward the ceiling, contracting your belly. Your tailbone and head curve toward the floor.

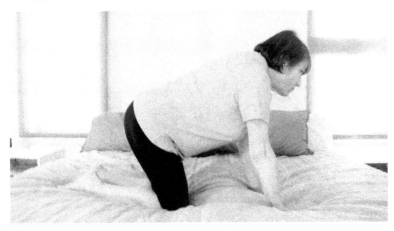

On inhalation, return to a flat back.

Repeat as many times as you like.

PILLOW-ASSISTED CHILD'S POSE

Restorative and relaxing, this pose stretches the spine, massages the internal organs, increases circulation to the head, and stimulates pituitary gland function. You may use a pillow to cushion your head.

Begin on your hands and knees.

Move your hips toward your heels, your chest and torso to your thighs, and your forehead to the floor (or pillow).

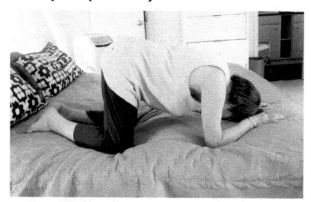

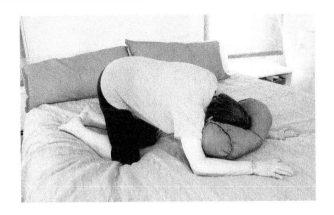

If this is uncomfortable, you may place a pillow between your torso and thighs, another behind your knees, a third under your ankles, and one for your head to rest on.

The entire body folds into a fetal position.

Stay until ready to resume yoga.

COBRA POSE

The Cobra Pose stretches the upper back, chest, and abdomen, stretches and relaxes the throat and shoulders, and strengthens the deep muscles of the spine.

Lie on your belly, place hands palm down under your shoulders alongside the chest.

On inhalation, expand your rib cage, lengthen your spine, draw your shoulders back and lift your head, neck, and chest slowly. The lift uses deep back muscles; the hands merely guide the position.

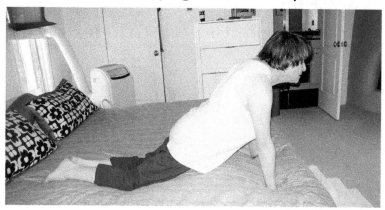

Breathe deeply.

Lift a little more with each inhalation over the course of 3 to 5 breaths.

BUTTERFLY POSE

The Butterfly Pose opens hips, stretches the groin, inner thighs, and knees.

From a seated position, bend your knees, and bring your heels in toward your sit bones.

Next, drop your knees out to the sides, press the soles of your feet together, and sit up as tall as you can, hands on feet or ankles.

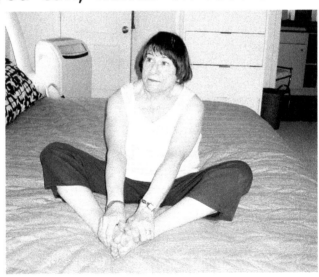

Let the weight of your legs gently open your hips.

Remain in position for 5 to 10 breaths.

SEATED MOUNTAIN

The Seated Mountain encourages awareness of the body and aids recognition and correction of any postural imbalances.

Sit in a chair, feet flat on the floor, back straight and not supported by the chair. For extra support, place a book or other flat, stable bolster under your feet.

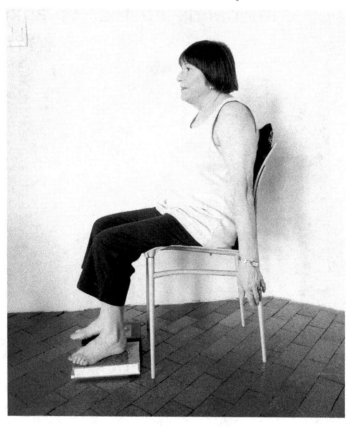

Tuck your chin and relax your shoulders.

Breathe deeply.

On an exhalation, press your feet into the floor, place your hands together in prayer position in front of your heart, and extend them over your head.

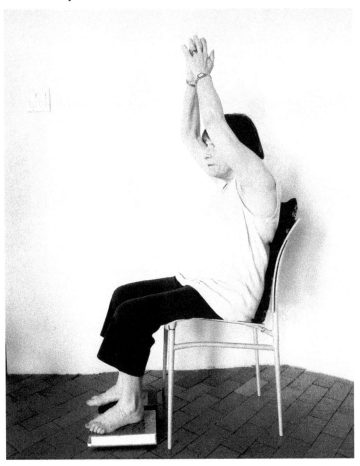

Notice the spine lengthening.

Stay as long as you wish, imagining yourself growing taller and taller.

SEATED FORWARD BEND

The Seated Forward Bend stretches and lengthens the spine, improving circulation and engaging the abdominal muscles.

Begin seated on a chair with feet flat on the floor (or sit as in Seated Mountain). Use a bolster or book under your feet for extra support.

Breathe deeply.

On an exhalation, fold forward as far as comfortable, bringing chest and belly toward thighs.

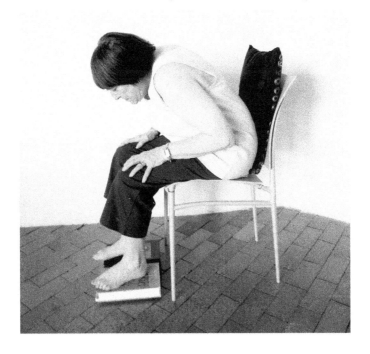

On inhalation, lift chest up away from thighs to return to a seated position.

Repeat 4 to 10 times.

SEATED FORWARD BEND WITH A STRAIGHT BACK

This pose encourages hip hinging to save the vertebrae from compression and improves flexibility in the hips.

Begin seated on a chair, feet flat on the floor (or sit as in Seated Mountain). Use a bolster under your feet for extra support.

Breathe deeply.

Keep the back straight as you exhale and fold as far forward as is comfortable. It helps to have the chin slightly tucked.

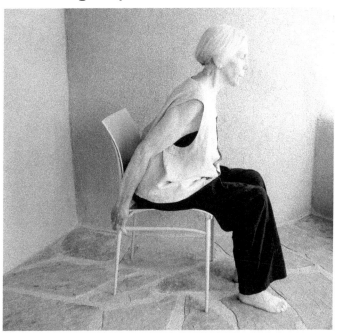

As you inhale, expand your chest, lengthen your spine and return to being seated upright. Repeat 4 to 10 times.

LATERAL NECK STRETCH

The Lateral Neck Stretch stretches and relaxes the lateral neck and upper shoulder muscles and improves circulation in the neck and shoulders.

Begin seated in a chair as in Seated Mountain. Use a bolster under your feet for extra support.

Drop your right ear toward your right shoulder.

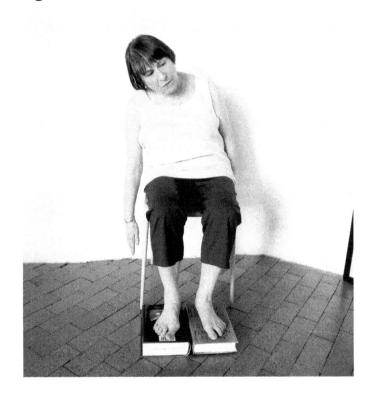

You may extend your hands toward the floor to further the

stretch and to be sure your shoulders do not rise up toward your ears.

Come back to center before repeating on the other side.

Be gentle.

SEATED HERO OR BREATH OF JOY

This pose increases energy, supports good posture, opens and expands the chest, and flattens and strengthens the upper back.

Begin seated in a chair as in Seated Mountain. Use a bolster under your feet for extra support.

Put your hands up, as if you are signaling "don't shoot."

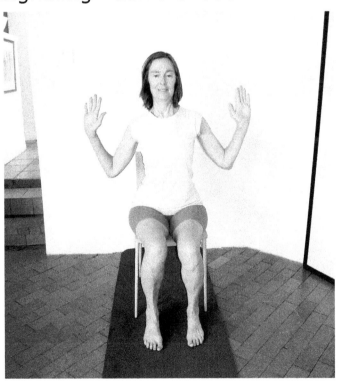

Breathe deeply.

Expand your chest on inhalation, opening arms wider.
Relax on exhalation.
Repeat for 5 to 10 breaths.

SEATED TWIST

The Seated Twist is calming and releases tension throughout the back. It stimulates the internal organs, improving digestion and elimination.

Sit as in Seated Mountain. Use a bolster under your feet for extra support.

Take your left arm to your right leg, and your right arm to the back of the chair.

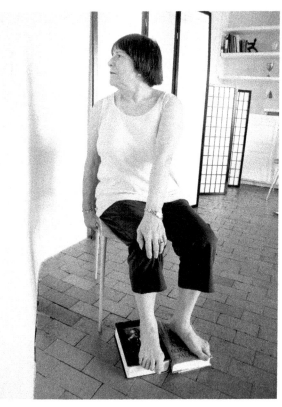

On inhalation, lengthen the front torso, from the belly up.

On exhalation, lean slightly back and turn your head right to complete the spinal twist, twisting from inside out. Continue to lengthen the spine, raising the ribs away from the pelvis and lifting the sternum with each inhalation, and twist a little more with each exhalation.

Repeat with each breath a few times before turning to do the same on the other side.

If you would like to intensify the twist, you may cross your legs, right over left if you are facing right.

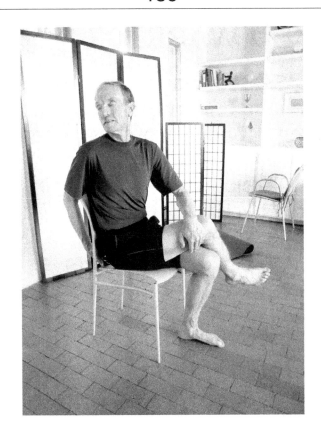

SEATED WARRIOR

The Seated Warrior brings flexibility to the spine muscles, tones the abdomen, and stretches the psoas muscle.

Sit sideways on a chair, extend your back leg behind, that is, to the right of the chair if you are facing left. It will seem as if you have only your left cheek on the chair.

Extend strongly through one or both arms at shoulder height.

Gaze forward, beyond your outstretched hand.

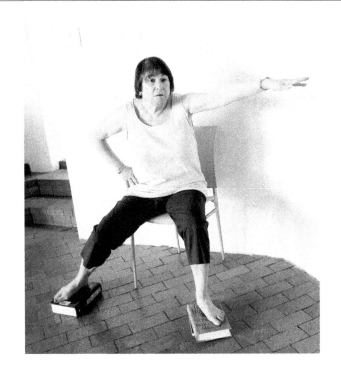

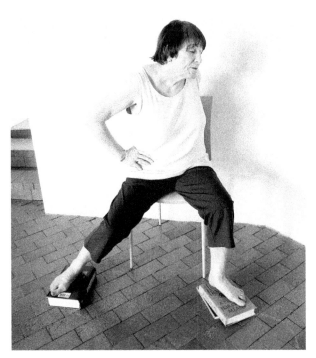

Alternatively, place hands on hips.

Stay a few breaths before doing the same on the second side.

CHAIR-ASSISTED CAMEL POSE

The Chair-Assisted Camel Pose stretches arms, upper back, and the entire torso. It relaxes the shoulders, opens the chest, and strengthens legs.

The Camel Pose is a kneeling backbend. Backbends are a great relief from desk work, computers, and everything that rounds us forward.

Kneel on the floor in front of a chair.

Place both hands on the chair behind you.

Press your hips forward as you look up, raise your chest, and drop your head back.

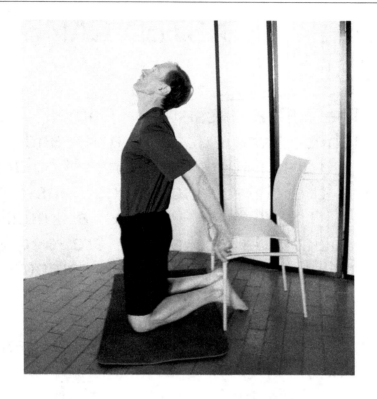

Stay for a few breaths.

10

Meditation

There are days when I find that just going out to lunch is a challenge worthy of King Arthur and all the knights of the roundtable. No telling when I'll feel up or down, on or off. As a fan of fairy tales, I liken myself to Cinderella, who one minute may be impeccably decked out (thanks to the assistance of the birds and creatures of the forest). Then, without any warning, I may find myself back on the mean streets, transformed into a ragamuffin pushing a pumpkin.

This is where meditation can be my Merlin. He offers me a way of dealing with the situation. There's no need to get depressed and have a pity-party when the magician can call upon my old reliable friends Theater of the Absurd and Sense of Humor to rescue me. Thanks to the meditative part of yoga (which my cats practice all the time), I can take a few minutes to calm my mind, which, and in turn, calms my body.

Simple yet profound, your ability to be fully present in the moment is one of the most beneficial practices in yoga.

You can meditate or pray in your very own individualistic way. As my creative writing teacher in college used to say about short stories: "Whatever works is right." With meditation, prayer, spiritualism, it has to work for you. One of the most unorthodox, creative interpreters of meditation is the writer Anne Lamott. In her book, *Help, Thanks, Wow,* Lamott quotes C.S. Lewis: "I pray because I can't help myself ... I pray because the need flows out of me all the time ... It doesn't change God. It changes me." Lamott continues this thought about how her spiritual practice helps her stay in the present moment, "More than anything, prayer (meditation) helps me get my sense of humor back. It brings me back to my heart ... it brings me back to the now, to the holy moment."

Yoga postures ground you in the body and help you to recognize areas of strength and weakness. Over time, the practices comprehensively promote overall health and well-being—mentally, emotionally, physically, and spiritually.

Meditation creates a time to listen to your inner voice, a voice that can help you make conscious choices about what is good, and not good, for your health. Meditation can also reduce stress, anxiety, worry, and depression.

For these reasons, I encourage a daily meditation practice:

- Set aside a time each day (mornings are often best, and an opportunity to "set the day in order").
- Choose a place that is quiet and uncluttered, where you will not be interrupted.
- Add a candle, flowers, music—anything to instill a feeling of beauty and peace.
- Make yourself comfortable, sitting or lying down.
- Slow your breathing and relax with the "observance of the breath" technique: in–pause–out.
- Ten to 20 minutes is a good beginning practice.

Do not put pressure on yourself to be perfect or create a rigid expectation about what meditating "should be." Let your practice unfold gently and naturally; be flexible; go where it takes you. Keep the daily practice going even when you feel discouraged, bored, or restless. The many benefits of meditation are experienced profoundly the longer one practices.

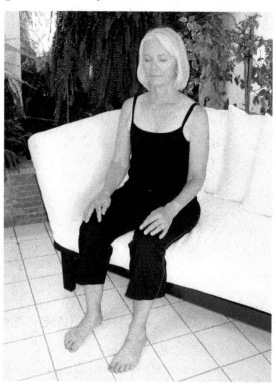

Conclusion

It is the artist's task to find out how much music you can still make with what you have left.
—Itzhak Perlman

One of my goals is to live a quality life with dignity for as long as I can. Exercise, and particularly yoga, helps me accomplish this goal. I'm not in perfect shape, but I want to do the most with what I have. I recently read an inspiring story in Dr. Larry Dossey's book *The Extraordinary Healing Power of Ordinary Things* about Itzhak Perlman, the famous violinist. It applies to us.

Perlman was stricken with polio as a child and walks with the aid of crutches and leg braces. When he comes onto the stage he has to make an enormous effort—putting his crutches down on the floor, unlocking his braces, tucking his feet just so, reaching for his violin before he can begin to play.

At a concert on November 18, 1995, things did not go smoothly for Perlman. After only a few bars of music, a violin string snapped with the sound of gunfire. The audience realized that the concert would have to pause for him to laboriously and painfully adjust his braces, pick up his crutches, walk off stage and repair the string or find another instrument. Instead, Perlman paused, closed his eyes and signaled the conductor to continue playing from where he left off.

As Rabbi Jack Reimer, who was present that night and related this account, said, "And he played with such passion and such power and such purity as we had never heard before. Of course, anyone knows that it is impossible to play a symphonic work with just three strings." I know that, and you know that, but that night Itzhak Perlman refused to know that. You could see him modulating, changing, recomposing the piece in his head. At one point, it sounded like he was de-tuning the strings to get new sounds from them that they had never made before.

When he was finished, the audience was stunned and rose to its feet, applauded and cheered. Reimer continues, "Then Perlman, smiled, wiped the sweat from his brow, raised his bow to quiet us and then he said, not boastfully, but in a quiet, pensive, reverent tone, *"You know sometimes it is the artist's task to find out how much music you can still make with what you have left."*"

That lovely sentiment is the underlying theme of this book—doing the most with what we have left.

That's what we all must strive to do.

Hope springs eternal—so get out your yoga mats!

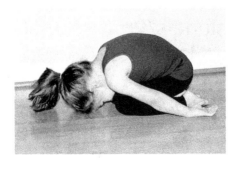

Notes

CHAPTER 2

[1]   p.14. *"According to a finding by the Parkinson's Foundation of the National Capital Area...":* parkinsonfoundation.org/yogaforparkinsons.html

[2]   p.14. *"A more academic study, performed by researchers at the JFK Institute in Denmark...":* T.W. Kjaer, C. Bertelsen, P. Piccini, D. Brooks, J. Alving, H.C. Lou. *Brain Research. Cognitive Brain Research* 13, no.2 (April 2002): 255–59.

[3]   p.14. *"I appreciate the better...":* positivehealth.com/article/yoga/yoga-for-parkinson-s

[4]   p.14. *"there is a growing body of evidence regarding the benefits of exercise...":* beta.parkinson.org/Professionals/Professionals---On-The-Blog/March-2010/Exercise-and-Parkinson-s-Disease

[5]   p.15. *"Yoga improves flexibility...":* www.guide4living.com/parkinsons/alternativetreatment

[6]   p.15. *"While exercise cannot cure this disease...":* Lori Newell. *The Book of Exercise and Yoga.* Charleston, SC.: BookSurge Publishing, 2005.

[7]   p.15. *"A surprising side effect was the social support...":* interview with author.

[8]   p.15. *"People with PD should have weekly Parkinson's exercise classes...":* interview with author.

CHAPTER 3

[1]   p.18. *"PD affects each person differently...":* Newell, *The Book of Exercise and Yoga.*

[2]   p.19. *"If you make the exercise grueling...":* John Argue. *Parkinson's Disease and The Art of Moving.* (Oakland, CA: New Harbinger Publications, 2000).

Resources

Parkinson's Disease Organizations

American Parkinson Disease Association
www.apdaparkinson.org
800-223-2732

National Parkinson Foundation
http://parkinson.org
800-473-4636

Parkinson's Action Network
www.parkinsonsaction.org
800-850-4726

Parkinson's Disease Foundation
www.pdf.org
800-457-6676

The Michael J. Fox Foundation
www.michaeljfox.org
800-708-7644

The Parkinson's Institute
www.thepi.org
800-655-2273

American Parkinson Disease Association
 National Young Onset Center
www.youngparkinsons.org
877-223-3801

Davis Phinney Foundation for Parkinson's
www.DavisPhinneyFoundation.org
866–358-0285

Northwest Parkinson's Foundation
www.nwpf.org
877-850-4726

Parkinson Alliance/Parkinson's Unity Walk
http://ParkinsonAlliance.org
800-579-8440

World Parkinson Congress
www.worldpdcongress.org
800.457.6676

Parkinson Society of Canada
Parkinson.Ca
800-565-3000

Parkinson's UK
www.parkinsons.org.uk
0808-800-0303

Parkinson Voice Project
http://ParkinsonVoiceProject.org
855-707-7325

OTHER HEALTH ORGANIZATIONS

American Association of People with
 Disabilities
http://aapd.com
800-840-8844

The Movement Disorder Society
www.movementdisorders.org
414-276-2145

National Institute of Neurological
 Disorders and Stroke
www.ninds.nih.gov
800-352-9424

PARKINSON'S DISEASE HEALTH CENTERS

Johns Hopkins Parkinson's Disease and
 Movement Disorders Center

www.hopkinsmedicine.org/neurology_ne urosurgery/specialty_areas/movement_ disorders

Parkinson's Disease and Movement Disorders Center, Northwestern University
www.parkinsons.northwestern.edu

PARKINSON'S REHABILITATION PROGRAMS

Neuro Fit
http://neuro-fit.com Lee Silverman Voice Treatment
www.lsvtglobal.com
888-438-5788

Lee Silverman Voice Treatment (LSVT) is a specific type of speech therapy tailored for people with PD. PD takes its toll on voices; 89 percent of people with PD have a problem with their speech and voice. Reduced loudness, monotone, hoarseness, and imprecise articulation are some of the most common characteristics. My speech mentor, the vivacious Cynthia Fox, vice president of Operations and cofounder, LSVT Global, Inc., who holds a PhD in speech pathology, has given me back my voice. Dr. Fox, who has enough energy to fuel a small nation, is a magician of sorts—she brings voices back to life.

YOGA FOR PD

National Parkinson Foundation: Yoga for Parkinson's at Kripalu Center for Yoga and Health
www.parkinson.org/Improving-Care/Education/Education--For-Patients/Wellness-Retreat-for-Recently-Diagnosed-Parkinsons

Duke Integrative Medicine – Therapeutic Yoga for Seniors professional training program
www.dukeintegrativemedicine.org

RECOMMENDED PARKINSON'S SUPPORT BOOKS

Argue, John. *Parkinson's Disease and the Art of Moving.* Oakland, CA: New Harbinger Publications, 2000. Argue is also the creator of a companion DVD, among other helpful resources. http://parkinsonsexercise.com

Newell, Lori. *The Book of Exercise and Yoga for Those with Parkinson's Disease: Using Movement and Meditation to Manage Symptoms.* Charleston, SC: BookSurge Publishing, 2005. Newell owns and operates Living Well Yoga and Fitness in the Hamptons. www.lwyf.org

YOGA ORGANIZATIONS

Kripalu Center for Yoga and Health
Stockbridge, MA
1-800-741-7353
http://kripalu.org

Paramahansa Yogananda's
 Self-Realization Fellowship
Los Angeles, CA
323-225-2471
www.yogananda-srf.org

American Viniyoga Institute
www.viniyoga.com

Iyengar Yoga
B.K.S. Iyengar Yoga National Association
 of the United States
http://iynaus.org

Yoga U
http://YogaUOnline.com

Yoga Anatomy
http://YogaAnatomy.net

International Association of Yoga
 Therapists
http://iayt.org

RECOMMENDED YOGA BOOKS

Desikachar, T.K.V. *The Heart of Yoga: Developing a Personal Practice.* Rochester, VT: Inner Traditions, 1999.

Kraftsow, Gary. *Yoga for Wellness: Healing with the Timeless Teachings of Viniyoga.* New York: Penguin, 1999.

Kraftsow, Gary. Yoga for Transformation: Ancient Teachings and Practices for Healing the Body, Mind, and Heart. New York: Penguin, 2002.

Coulter, H. David. *Anatomy of Hatha Yoga: A Manual for Students, Teachers, and Practitioners.* Indianapolis: Body and Breath, 2010.

Faulds, Richard, and Senior Teachers of Kripalu Center for Yoga and Health. *Kripalu Yoga: A Guide to Practice On and Off the Mat.* New York: Bantam Dell, 2006.

Carrico, Mara, and the editors of *Yoga Journal. Yoga Journal's Yoga Basics. New York:* Henry Holt, 1997.

Ansari, Mark, and Liz Lark. *Yoga for Beginners.* New York: William Morrow, 1999.

Yee, Rodney. *Yoga: The Poetry of the Body: A 50-Card Practice Deck. New York: St.* Martin's Griffin, 2003.

Falloon-Goodhew, Peter. *Stay Young: Yoga for Living. New York: D.K. Publishing, Inc.,* 2002.

Rappaport, Julie. *365 Yoga: Daily Meditations. New York: Jeremy P. Tarcher/Penguin,* 2004.

YOGA PERIODICALS

Yoga Journal
415-591-0555
www.yogajournal.com

YOGA Magazine
www.yogamagazine.com

Rivington House
82 Great Eastern Street
London EC2A 3JF

Flow, Yoga Magazine
www.flowyogamagazine.com

Yoga International
www.himalayaninstitute.org/yoga-intern
 ational-magazine/

Yogi Times
www.yogitimes.com/
310.439.9583
PO Box 5153
Santa Monica, CA 90409-5153

RECOMMENDED BOOKS FOR IMPROVING POSTURE

Gokhale, Ester. *8 Steps to a Pain Free Back: Natural Posture Solutions for Pain in the Back, Neck, Shoulder, Hip, Knee, and Foot.* Chicago: Pendo Press, 2008.

Meeks, Sara. *WALK TALL! An Exercise Program for the Prevention and Treatment of Back Pain, Osteoporosis and the Postural Changes of Aging.* Gainsville, FL: Triad Publishing, 2010.

COMPLEMENTARY MODALITIES

Acupuncture
Doctors Jason Jishun and Linda Lingzhi
 Hao (in Santa Fe, NM)
Hao and Hao
505-986-0542

Southwest Acupuncture College
www.acupuncturecollege.edu
505-438-8884

Reiki
http://ilovereiki.com

Angela and Karl Robb, Reiki Masters
www.GiveReiki.com
Specializing in Reiki for Parkinson's and
 Parkinson's Caregivers nationwide.

Back Cover Material

Ease stiffness, improve strength and balance, and relieve stress with gentle, easy yoga postures

Yoga is one of the most beneficial complementary therapies for Parkinson's disease (PD), helping to increase flexibility, correct posture, loosen tight, painful muscles, build confidence, and in general, enhance the quality of life. Peggy van Hulsteyn, who was diagnosed with PD 12 years ago, has experienced these benefits firsthand. In *YOGA AND PARKINSON'S DISEASE,* van Hulsteyn draws on her 40-year yoga practice, collaborating with two certified yoga teachers, to provide an accessible, easy-to-follow, and encouraging guide for bringing the benefits of yoga into your life, even if you've never done yoga before.

YOGA AND PARKINSON'S DISEASE includes:

- Step-by-step instructions and easy-to-follow photographs

- Seated and assisted postures for those with limited mobility or unsteadiness
- Postures that can be done in bed to help you start your day
- Variations to ensure comfort and safety
- Tips for making yoga practice easy, approachable, and sustainable, and much more.

***

"With compassion, humor, and a hard-fought perspective, van Hulsteyn has written an inspiring book and seeks to provide a practical guide to others in coping with Parkinson's disease."
—U.S. SENATOR TOM UDALL (D-NM)

"A must-read.... Her practical tips and well-explained poses will help anyone with Parkinson's explore ways to live as fully as possible."
—JOYCE OBERDORF, president and CEO, National Parkinson Foundation

***

Peggy van Hulsteyn is an accomplished author and speaker who has practiced yoga for over four decades. She was diagnosed with Parkinson's disease 12 years ago. Since then, she has devoted her talents and energy to improving the lives of those with PD. Her cover article for *Yoga Journal* on the tangible benefits yoga can bring to people with PD drew international acclaim. She and her physicist husband, David, divide their time between Santa Fe, New Mexico and Tucson, Arizona. Visit her at www.pdhatlady.com

Barbara Gage is a certified Kripalu Yoga teacher. She has been a yoga teacher for 35 years and is a respected psychotherapist in private practice. She lives in Santa Fe, New Mexico. www.barbaragage.com

Connie Fisher is certified in yoga therapy from the American Viniyoga Institute in California. She is also a doctor of Oriental medicine and a massage therapist. She lives in Seattle, Washington.